Bath University Library

28 DAY LOAN

This book should be returned not later than the last date stamped below. The period of loan may be extended on request if no other reader wishes to use the book. **Books may not be renewed by telephone.**

If this book is reserved by another reader it will be recalled and must be returned by the date on the recall notice, or fines will be incurred.

Cover design: The black pyramid represents the population of Western Europe in 1975 (males on the left, females on the right) and the red pyramid the same population in 2000.

World Health Organization
Regional Office for Europe
Copenhagen

Demographic trends in the European Region

Health and social implications

Edited by

Alan D. Lopez

Global Epidemiological Surveillance and Health Situation Assessment
World Health Organization
Geneva

and

Robert L. Cliquet

Centre for Population and Family Studies
Brussels

WHO Regional Publications, European Series No. 17

The WHO Regional Office for Europe
wishes to express its gratitude to
the United Nations Fund for Population Activities
for financially supporting this work
under project RMI/79/P05

ISBN 92 890 1108 4

CONTENTS

PART III — HEALTH AND SOCIAL IMPLICATIONS

PART IV — CONCLUSIONS AND RECOMMENDATIONS

Foreword

In May 1977, the Thirtieth World Health Assembly resolved that "the main social target of governments and WHO in the coming decades should be the attainment by all citizens of the world by the year 2000 of a level of health that will permit them to lead a socially and economically productive life". In Europe, the meaning of that goal was further developed in the regional strategy for attaining health for all by the year 2000, adopted by the WHO Regional Committee for Europe in 1980. The translation of policy statements and strategies into effective programmes aiming at specific targets has started in several countries, as well as in WHO. The success of the entire enterprise depends on the relevance of choices made now, based on proper assessments and forecasts of needs and resources. At least three basic issues are involved in the long-term planning for health for all. First, we should define what level of health we expect to attain, in terms of reducing negative aspects —premature death, disease, disability — and enhancing positive aspects. Second, we should say how we intend to attain this level of health, by promoting lifestyles conducive to health, reducing risks, and developing adequate health care. Third, we must have the best possible knowledge of the population involved, in terms of numbers, structure and dynamics. For all three issues, knowledge of trends is essential in providing the background for projections and forecasts.

Among a series of efforts aimed at improving knowledge in this field the Regional Office, with the active support of the United Nations Fund for Population Activities, initiated in 1980 a study on the health and social implications of trends in demographic structure. It is my hope that the results of that study, as presented here, will help those responsible for preparing for the future within their own countries to understand better the complex interrelations between health status, social and economic factors, and demographic change. I hope, too, that this book will enable them to identify the best ways of coping with such change in order to ensure the health and wellbeing of the entire population.

Leo A. Kaprio

WHO Regional Director for Europe

Acknowledgements

The Study on Demographic Trends in the European Region: Health and Social Implications was a joint effort of the WHO Regional Office for Europe, the United Nations Fund for Population Activities and several national health authorities, experts and institutions.

The Regional Office would like to thank the following for their valuable contributions:

- the health authorities of the 15 countries that submitted national reports, namely Algeria, Belgium, Czechoslovakia, the German Democratic Republic, Finland, Greece, Hungary, Luxembourg, Monaco, Morocco, the Netherlands, Norway, Portugal, Switzerland and the United Kingdom;

- the participants in the meeting organized in Berne in March 1982 (see Annex 1);

- the editors of the present report and the authors of working documents;

- the members of the Steering Group:

  Professor Z. Brzeziński, Poland
  Professor R.L. Cliquet, Belgium
  Professor A.J. Fox, United Kingdom
  Professor E. Heikkinen, Finland
  Dr A. Klinger, Hungary
  Ms E. Lynge, Denmark
  Dr P. Paillat, France
  Ms S. Teper, United Kingdom

- the federal authorities of Switzerland, who hosted the meeting, and especially Dr U. Frey, Director of the Federal Office of Public Health and Mr J.J. Senglet, Director of the Federal Statistical Office.

Introduction

A.D. Lopez & R.L. Cliquet

The World Health Organization's regional strategies for attaining the goal of health for all closely reflect the nature of the most common health problems found in the respective regions. In the European Region, where the majority of countries have completed the mortality transition and where the profile of ill health is dominated by the chronic diseases, the strategy focuses on promoting lifestyles conducive to health, reducing preventable conditions, and reorienting the health care system to better serve the needs of the entire population.

A critical element in the implementation of this strategy is the process of demographic change. Thus the demand for health services in future will to a considerable extent be determined by changes in population structure, since the risks of suffering ill health are closely related to such demographic characteristics as age, sex, social class and place of residence. Similarly, changes in fertility, in family formation and in the propensity to migrate will affect a host of health and social services.

In an endeavour to anticipate such changing needs, the WHO Regional Office for Europe initiated a project in 1980 to study demographic change in the Region with a view to providing the necessary background information for the regional strategy. More specifically, the major objectives of the study were to:

— assess changes in demographic structure with reference to social and economic roles and functions of population groups in countries with different patterns of population dynamics and development;

— examine the way in which different countries cope with such changes and the measures they employ to secure the development and wellbeing of the total population, and in particular of vulnerable groups; and

— make recommendations on developing health, social and related services according to the population needs arising from such demographic changes.

At the same time, a parallel project on projections of the future health situation in Europe is being undertaken to predict the development of health status and its implications for health and social services.

On the recommendations of a planning meeting convened in Copenhagen in 1980, the Regional Office, in cooperation with the Government of Switzerland and with the support of the United Nations Fund for Population Activities (UNFPA), organized a technical meeting on trends in demographic structure in the European Region, in Berne in March 1982. The meeting was attended by delegates from Belgium, Finland, France, the Federal Republic of Germany, Greece, Hungary, the Netherlands, Poland, Portugal, Sweden, Switzerland and the United Kingdom. Representatives of the Commission of the European Communities (CEC), the Council of Europe (CE), the United Nations Economic Commission for Europe (ECE), UNFPA and the International Institute for Applied Systems Analysis (IIASA) were also present.

Following the opening session, six working papers were presented on demographic trends in the European Region with regard to fertility, family formation and mortality, and on the effects of these trends on young people, adults and the elderly, with particular reference to health and social policy. Fourteen country reports were also available, of which a synopsis was presented. Subsequently, the participants separated into three working groups to formulate conclusions and recommendations with respect to the topics identified during the preceding sessions. The working groups focused on issues of concern to each of the three broad age groups: 0–19 years, 20–59 years, and 60 years and over. The reports of the three working groups were then discussed in plenary, leading to the conclusions and recommendations presented in Chapter 8 of this book. As a general point, it may be mentioned here that while this age division was considered preferable for the purposes of the study, it was not always possible to adhere to it in the working papers owing to the preference for other age groupings in many of the studies cited. This is particularly true for the elderly, where the age group 65 years and over is frequently used.

The working papers for the meeting are presented in Parts I, II and III of the book. Part I provides an overview of demographic change in the Region and its more important health and social consequences, based on the 14 country reports prepared for the study. What is abundantly clear from this synopsis is that, while the extent and timing of changes in fertility, mortality and migration have varied markedly from one country to another, the consequences of these changes are remarkably similar for most countries and will become even more so as the various Member States move towards greater demographic uniformity.

Part II deals with the analysis of recent demographic trends in the European Region. In Chapter 2, a number of significant developments in family formation and dissolution are outlined, prominent among them being the trend towards postponement of first marriage, the rising proportion of single-person households, and the increasing propensity for marriage to end in divorce. Trends of fertility in Europe, which are strongly dependent on these changes in family formation, are discussed in the next chapter. Not only has there been a marked reduction in average completed family size in most countries, but also the period of childbearing has contracted, with the result that births to older women are becoming increasingly rare. The trend towards increasing life expectancy in Europe is discussed in Chapter 4. What is particularly impressive about recent mortality changes in the Region is the diversity of country experience. This is most evident among adult males. Indeed, in the Northern European countries life expectancy for men remained roughly constant during the 1960s and 1970s, and has even declined in parts of Eastern Europe over the last decade or so. At the same time, persistent differentials in survival are evident among population subgroups. These are perhaps best documented according to social and/or occupational class, with the poor being the most vulnerable. An important challenge for future research into differentials in ill health will be to determine to what extent this is a reflection of less healthy lifestyles, of greater occupational hazards, or of less efficacious use of health services, and to guide the reorientation of health education programmes and health services accordingly.

The process of demographic change does not, of course, occur in a vacuum, and as such is likely to have profound health and social consequences. These are examined in Part III according to broad life-cycle stages. With infant and child mortality already at very low levels throughout much of the Region, the principal issues of concern for the young population are now related more to changes in sexual behaviour and abortion among adolescents and other aspects of psychosocial development. Among adults on the other hand, the trend towards smaller family and household size, coupled with increasing divorce rates, will further increase the number of adults living in isolation. Certainly, traditional health and social services, as well as housing policy, will need to be more flexible to meet the special requirements of this group. Greater flexibility in working conditions, including such measures as job sharing, will also be necessary to allow couples more freedom in deciding on their respective economic participation and its timing during working life. Sustained periods of unemployment are also of considerable concern for many in this age group, requiring a more comprehensive and concerted approach by health, social and political institutions to deal effectively with its consequences.

However, perhaps the most significant demographic change to have occurred in the European Region, over the last few decades at least, has been the dramatic aging of the population with marked increases in the number and proportion of the elderly in most countries. Moreover, there is every reason to believe that this trend will continue into the twenty-first century, carrying with it a host of implications for the support services. This may well require that long-term health care programmes be "de-institutionalized" and provide for more independent alternative living arrangements for the individual. Simultaneously, home health care services will need to be better developed, requiring in many instances a reorientation of the role of the family in the care of the aged. But perhaps of equal importance is the challenge of providing creative vocational opportunities for the elderly, thereby encouraging their further self-development.

In attempting to highlight the major demographic trends in the Region and their implications for health and social services, it is inevitable that the book will only touch on many issues that deserve far greater attention and which are likely to become of increasing concern. A number of less favourable developments commensurate with modern technology and rapid social change are only now emerging, and knowledge about their effects on health is still comparatively embryonic. Thus the "chemicalization" of society may well be as yet too recent a phenomenon for significant health consequences to be demonstrated. The substantial progress in reducing early infant and fetal mortality has increased the need for sophisticated postnatal equipment to sustain those infants who would previously have succumbed to congenital infirmities or birth injuries. By the same token, the lengthening of life may not always be accompanied by a reduction of morbidity, which would permit the elderly to enjoy more years of healthy life and thereby diminish their requirements for specialized and expensive health care. These and indeed many of the issues discussed in the following pages emphasize the need for greater interdisciplinary cooperation among demographers, epidemiologists and others concerned with population change and its consequences. For it is only through such enhanced cooperation that the admirable health goals of the Region can be attained.

Part I

Synopsis
of country reports

1

Demographic change in Europe and its health and social implications: an overview[a]

A.D. Lopez

The principal elements of the strategy of the European Region of WHO for achieving health for all by the year 2000 include the promotion of lifestyles conducive to health, the reduction of preventable conditions, and the provision of adequate and accessible health care. Of the many factors that influence the design and implementation of programmes to achieve these aims, population structure and the components of demographic change are of major importance. Investigations of the health situation have invariably shown that the nature and extent of ill health differs widely among population subgroups. The representation of these groups in the total population depends, in turn, on previous levels and trends of fertility, mortality and geographical mobility.

Even within such a comparatively demographically homogeneous region as Europe, where most countries have long since completed the process of demographic transition, significant intercountry and, indeed, intracountry variations in demographic behaviour are to be found. To attain the health goals of the Region, these differences must be recognized and appropriate emphasis given to assessing their significance in relation to the overall regional strategy. With this in mind, the 33 Member States of the Region were invited to prepare an analysis of their demographic situation and to comment on the major health and social implications arising from it. Reports were received from 15 countries: Algeria, Belgium, Czechoslovakia, Finland, the German Democratic Republic, Greece, Hungary, Luxembourg, Monaco,[b] Morocco, the Netherlands, Norway, Portugal, Sweden and the United Kingdom (Great Britain). Whilst the reports provided comprehensive analyses of demographic trends, much less attention was paid to the health and social consequences arising from them. In this chapter

[a] The author is indebted to Dr Lene Mikkelsen, who helped considerably in the preparation of an earlier draft of this paper, and to Ms Sue Teper for her many helpful comments on it.

[b] Given the small population size of the Principality, the number of demographic events (births, deaths, migrations) is insufficient to permit statistically reliable comparisons.

a synthesis of the major findings of these country reports will be presented in conjunction with other, more global analyses of demographic phenomena in Europe.[a] In this way, the individual country situation can be placed in the broader perspective of a general overview of demographic change in the Region.

The first part of the chapter is devoted to a review of earlier demographic trends. These are considered under the separate components of demographic change: population growth and structure, family formation, fertility, mortality and population movement. The implications of these trends are considered in the second part of the chapter, drawing, whenever possible, on the actual projections presented in many of the country reports.

Recent Demographic Trends in the European Region

Population growth and composition

The size of a population as well as its composition depends on previous levels of and trends in fertility, mortality and population movement. Differentials in these determinants between population subgroups are of particular importance. Population size and structure, therefore, are often viewed as the intermediate variables between the basic processes of demographic change and the social, economic, public health and other consequences of this change. In this respect, population growth and composition may be considered as a "summary indicator" of previous demographic trends.

Regional trends

An overview of population change in the European Region over the last three decades is given in Table 1. This shows average growth rates for the major geographical subdivisions[b] according to broad age groups. As might be expected, the highest population growth has occurred in the less developed countries of the Region — Algeria, Morocco and Turkey — where total population size has increased by approximately 30% in each decade between 1950 and 1980. Similarly, the pattern of change for the various age groups in these three countries shows a remarkable degree of internal consistency, albeit at different levels of population growth. In general, the population of children and young people (0–19 years) has continued to grow at a rate comparable to that of the total population, whereas the growth rate of the working age population (20–59 years) declined in all three countries during the 1960s, only to rise again during the 1970s. Conversely, population growth among the elderly (60 and over) tended to increase during the 1960s, with the exception of Turkey. Since then, it has fallen dramatically, especially in Morocco.

[a] A preliminary synthesis of the country reports was prepared by Z. Brzeziński for the meeting in Berne in 1982. Additional country reports were subsequently received and have been included in the present study.

[b] For the country composition of these geographical divisions, see the note to Table 1.

Table 1. Decennial rates of population growth in the European Region by age and major geographical division, 1950–1980

Country or region[a]	Percentage change in population size											
	All ages			Ages 0–19			Ages 20–59			Ages 60+		
	1950–1960	1960–1970	1970–1980	1950–1960	1960–1970	1970–1980	1950–1960	1960–1970	1970–1980	1950–1960	1960–1970	1970–1980
Eastern Europe	9.3	6.8	6.5	8.2	2.8	- 3.3	6.2	3.7	14.0	27.7	30.7	3.6
Northern Europe	4.6	5.9	2.0	8.7	6.3	- 4.6	- 0.4	1.9	3.4	14.9	18.1	9.8
Southern Europe	8.8	8.1	8.9	1.9	6.9	2.4	11.0	4.5	11.1	21.8	27.1	16.4
Western Europe	9.9	10.1	3.0	10.8	12.4	- 6.5	6.2	4.6	10.0	21.5	23.4	0.1
USSR	19.0	13.8	9.3	10.1	17.2	- 3.0	23.6	10.0	15.6	32.9	21.6	22.9
Algeria	23.4	23.2	39.7	31.9	34.5	39.8	16.2	6.6	43.8	6.2	34.6	16.5
Morocco	30.0	29.9	34.2	31.2	34.7	34.5	29.1	17.5	38.6	23.2	85.7	4.9
Turkey	32.2	28.4	28.4	31.7	34.4	22.8	31.1	20.4	37.1	45.0	36.9	18.4

[a] Regions as defined by the United Nations. *Eastern Europe* includes Bulgaria, Czechoslovakia, the German Democratic Republic, Hungary, Poland and Romania; *Northern Europe* includes the Channel Islands, Denmark, the Faroe Islands, Finland, Iceland, Ireland, the Isle of Man, Norway, Sweden and the United Kingdom; *Southern Europe* includes Albania, Andorra, Gibraltar, Greece, the Holy See, Italy, Malta, Portugal, San Marino, Spain and Yugoslavia; *Western Europe* includes Austria, Belgium, France, the Federal Republic of Germany, Liechtenstein, Luxembourg, Monaco, the Netherlands and Switzerland.

Source: Computed from *World population and its age–sex composition by country, 1950–2000: demographic estimation and projection as assessed in 1978*. New York, United Nations Population Division, Department of Economic and Social Affairs, 1981.

Undoubtedly, one of the most important features demonstrated in Table 1 is the rapid growth of the elderly population throughout Europe and the USSR during the 1950s and 1960s. Typically, the rate of population increase for this age group was about 10–20% higher than that for the younger ages. During the 1970s, however, there was a marked deceleration in population growth among the elderly in some regions — notably in Western Europe, where the size of this group has effectively remained unchanged, but also in Eastern Europe where only marginal growth has occurred. Conversely, the population of working age increased much more rapidly during the 1970s (compared with the two earlier decades) in all regions.

Equally impressive is the dramatic decline in population growth over the last two decades for the group aged 0–19 years. In the USSR, for example, the population at these ages fell by 3% during the 1970s, having grown by more than 17% during the 1960s. Indeed, in all the regions of Europe — with the exception of the southernmost part — the numbers of children and adolescents have fallen over the last ten years as a result of a decline in fertility.

Perhaps a more convenient index for assessing these changes in population structure is to examine trends in the dependency ratios. These express the young, the old, and the combined young and old populations as a ratio of the population of working age. Some ratios are shown in Table 2. The relative aging of the population in the Region is obvious from the general trend towards increasing old-age dependency ratios. This is particularly evident for countries in Northern Europe where the old-age dependency ratio increased monotonically from 27 per 100 persons of working age in 1950 to almost 40 per 100 in 1980. A similar trend in this ratio is also apparent for Southern Europe. However, one should also note that a decline occurred in the old-age dependency ratio during the 1970s in Eastern and Western Europe as well as in the less developed countries of the Region. This reflects the relatively rapid growth of the working age population in these areas during that period.

The demographic impact of high fertility is evident from the comparatively high child dependency ratios observed in Algeria, Morocco and Turkey. Moreover, the ratios in these countries show a rapid increase between 1950 and 1970, although since that date a noticeable decline has occurred. From Table 1 it is apparent that the reduction in these ratios in recent years is largely a reflection of the rapid expansion in the adult population (that is, in the denominator of the ratio). In Turkey a sizeable decline in population growth at the younger ages has made an additional contribution to the decline. Of the four geographical regions of the Continent, only in Southern Europe has the child dependency ratio declined more or less monotonically over the period.

Country change

This broad overview of regional population change provides a useful background against which to evaluate trends in individual countries. In the two countries of Southern Europe for which reports were received, the early 1970s

Table 2. Age dependency ratios in the European Region, 1950–1980

Country or region[a]	Child dependency ratio[b]				Old-age dependency ratio[c]			
	1950	1960	1970	1980	1950	1960	1970	1980
Eastern Europe	0.66	0.67	0.67	0.57	0.20	0.24	0.31	0.28
Northern Europe	0.55	0.60	0.62	0.58	0.27	0.31	0.36	0.39
Southern Europe	0.72	0.66	0.67	0.62	0.21	0.23	0.28	0.30
Western Europe	0.56	0.59	0.63	0.54	0.27	0.31	0.37	0.33
USSR	0.78	0.69	0.74	0.62	0.18	0.19	0.21	0.22
Algeria	1.16	1.32	1.67	1.62	0.16	0.14	0.18	0.15
Morocco	1.35	1.37	1.57	1.52	0.08	0.11	0.17	0.13
Turkey	1.12	1.13	1.26	1.13	0.13	0.15	0.17	0.15

[a] For the United Nations definition of European regions see Table 1.

[b] Ratio of population aged 0–19 to that aged 20–59.

[c] Ratio of population aged 60+ to that aged 20–59.

Source: Computed from *World population and its age-sex composition by country, 1950–2000: demographic estimation and projection as assessed in 1978*, New York, United Nations Population Division, Department of Economic and Social Affairs, 1981.

were characterized by rapid population expansion. Between 1970 and 1975 the average annual population growth rate in Portugal was of the order of 1.35%, due primarily to the return of Portuguese nationals from former African colonies and to a decline in emigration from Portugal. In Greece, too, the 10.7% increase in population during the 1970s largely reflected migration gains. Over the last 20 years population growth in Greece has averaged around 0.7% per year. The most significant structural change in this country has been the increase in the proportion of people aged 60 and over from 8.2% in 1961 to 10.9% in 1981. This population "aging" has been more marked in the rural areas, where the proportion of those aged 60 and over has increased from 8.8% to 12.8%. Another interesting feature of population change in Greece is the decline in the proportion classified as illiterate. Between 1961 and 1971 this proportion fell by about one fifth to 14% of the total population aged 10 years and over — although, as one might expect, the decline in the rural areas was more moderate (a fall of roughly one eighth). During the 1960s there was a noticeable decline in the proportion of the population aged 10 or over who were economically active (from 54% to 46%). According to the Greek report, there is a certain consistency between these developments in that the latter decline in labour force participation can be ascribed to an increase in school enrolments, and to the advent of social reforms precluding or discouraging labour among young children and the aged.

A significant feature of population change in the German Democratic Republic has been the decline in total population size since the end of the 1960s. In 1970, for example, the population of the country stood at 17 075 000. By 1975 this had declined by 184 000, and the number had fallen by a further 151 000 by 1980. According to the German report, a lower birth rate together with increasing mortality contributed to this situation. On the other hand in Hungary, where mortality has also been rising in recent years, the population grew by about 3.5% during each of the two decades 1960–1970 and 1970–1980. The population pyramids of both the German Democratic Republic and Hungary, however, have been markedly affected by the two world wars. In the German Democratic Republic this has resulted in a relatively high proportion of the population (16%) being aged 65 and over. Similarly, the number of people aged 50–54 in Hungary is currently about two thirds higher than it was in 1970 owing to a fall in birth rate during the First World War. One consequence of the aging of these small birth cohorts is the stabilization in the proportion of the population aged 60 and over between 1970 and 1980. More specifically, the number of persons aged 60–64 in 1980 was about one third less than in 1970. However, over the same period those aged 65 and over had increased by 22% and those aged 75 and over by about one third. Much the same development, an "aging" of the aging population so to speak, is also evident in the German Democratic Republic.

A noticeable trend towards urbanization can be seen for the Eastern European countries. In Czechoslovakia the trend is apparent throughout the period 1960–1980. It has been particularly pronounced in the Slovak Socialist Republic, with the result that the urbanization gap between the two constituent republics has diminished. In 1961 some 30.5% of the population in the Czech Socialist Republic lived in communities of 20 000 or more, compared with 13.6% in the Slovak Socialist Republic. By 1979 the proportions had increased to 39.7% and 30.3% respectively, and 36.6% for the country as a whole. In the German Democratic Republic the rise from 22.0% to 25.9% in the proportion of the population living in cities of 100 000 or more between 1970 and 1980 appears to have occurred at the expense of those living in small communities of fewer than 1000 inhabitants. There has, however, been little change in the share of the total accounted for by those living in communities of 1000–5000 persons (currently about one fifth). A similar exodus to the urban centres has occurred in Hungary. Between 1960 and 1980 the proportion living in rural areas in Hungary declined from 55.7% to 46.8%, with a corresponding increase in the population living in urban areas other than the capital. Interestingly, few of those leaving the rural districts appear to have moved to Budapest.

A good description of the consequences of social and demographic change, at least for the economically active population in Hungary, is given in the country report. Commenting on the decline in both the number and proportion of the working population in the 1970s, the report attributes this to the fact that over the last decade:

> No significant mobilizable labour reserve was available, smaller and smaller age-groups entered the productive age and ... of them many continued [at school] so [that] the replacement of youth decreased gradually. At the same time the number and proportion of old people grew and as [pension schemes became more accessible] the share of pensioners continued to increase. The spread of [retirement exemptions with age], the gradual decrease of the [retirement] age [for] members of farmers' co-operatives as well as the greater utilization of the child care allowance contributed to the decrease in employment.

The impact of two world wars on the population pyramids is also evident for the countries of Western Europe. In both Belgium and Luxembourg the indentations at ages 35–39 and 60–64 years reflect the lower fertility of couples during the First and Second World War, respectively. The consequences of "la grande crise" for population structure in Luxembourg are also clear from the pyramid — with the smaller birth cohorts of the 1930s. Furthermore, as the Belgian report notes, the symmetry of population composition in the European Region is aggravated by the differential mortality of the sexes, with an over-representation of older women in the population because of their more favourable survival chances. The progressive impact of this factor on population structure is well documented in the Netherlands report. The latest population figures for this country reveal a 10% excess of females at ages 65–69, increasing to 24% at ages 70–74 and to 36% at ages 75–79, and reaching 50% at ages 80–84. At younger ages, however, the surplus of males arising from the predominance of male births is being extended to higher and higher ages. Thus in 1960 the deficit of females in the Netherlands continued up to age 30. Since then there has been a progressive rise in the age at which the imbalance of the sexes is reversed so that by 1980, the deficit of females was still apparent up to the age of 50 years.

The significance of migration for population growth in some countries of Western Europe is best exemplified by Luxembourg. Since 1967 the number of Luxembourgeois has been declining on average by about 1000 per year as a consequence of the older age structure of the population.[a] Overall, however, the population has increased from 340 000 in 1970 to 365 000 in 1980 because of an influx of immigrants, especially from Portugal. Immigrants have also accounted for much of the population growth in the Netherlands since 1970. During the decade 1960–1969 only about 5.5% of total population growth was due to migration gains; during the 1970s a rise in immigration, together with a roughly constant emigration rate, accounted for almost one third of population increase. At the same time

[a] An older population will *inter alia* lead to a rise in the number of deaths because of a much higher probability of death at the older ages. This is likely to be of particular significance for Luxembourg which, according to the country report, has the oldest age structure in the world.

there have been a number of significant changes in population distribution within the Netherlands. Between 1960 and 1980 the proportion of the population residing in municipalities of 100 000 or more declined from about one third to a little over one quarter. Over the same period the proportion living in towns of fewer than 5000 declined by about half to account for about 5% of the total population in 1980. Conversely, the share of the population living in municipalities of 20 000–50 000 grew from around 15% to 25% of the population by 1980. One consequence of this trend has been the more rapid aging of the urban population: 13% of those living in large towns and cities in the Netherlands in 1980 were aged 65 and over, compared with only 9% of those living in municipalities of 5000–50 000.

However, perhaps nowhere in Europe is the phenomenon of population aging as advanced as it is in Scandinavia where, for many years, adult mortality rates were the lowest in the world. In Norway, for example, the size of the population aged 70 and over has increased by 60% in the last 20 years, compared with an increase of only 14% for the total population. Over the same period the proportion of the Swedish population aged 65 and over has grown from 12% to 16.4% of the total. Furthermore, the number aged 80 and above increased by almost 40% during the 1970s, the vast majority of them women.

In addition, a number of alterations to the pattern of labour force participation have taken place which have had, and will continue to have, important implications for the organization of health and social services. Of major importance is the increasing participation in economic activities outside the home of married women. Between 1960 and 1970 in Norway, for example, the proportion of married women working increased from 10% to 23%, rising further to 58% in 1980. Moreover, this trend is evident in all age groups between 20 and 59 years. There has been a rise in the female workforce in Finland in recent decades, which has largely offset the decline in the proportion of males who are economically active.[a] Concurrent with this development, in Finland (as elsewhere) a reduction in employment in agriculture and forestry has occurred. In 1960 some 35% of the economically active population in Finland were occupied in these industries; by 1975 this proportion had declined to 15% with, of course, a corresponding increase in the workforce engaged in the professional, technical and administrative categories.

The phenomenon of population aging is unquestionably one of the most significant demographic features of the European Region during the last quarter century. The characteristics and extent of the trend have, of course, varied from one country to another reflecting earlier demographic history. A concise description of the process in Great Britain, as well as its causes and consequences, is to be found in the country report. In so far as the process in Britain is broadly representative of the development in other countries, it is worth quoting from the report in full:

---

[a] From 57.5% of the adult male population in 1960 to 51.7% in 1975.

... one of the most important changes in the age distribution during the last 25 years has been the increase, both in absolute numbers and as a proportion of the population, of the elderly. The number of persons of pensionable age (men aged 65 and over and women aged 60 and over) has risen by over 40 percent from 6.7 million in 1951 to 9.4 million in 1976. As a proportion of the total population this group has increased from nearly 14 percent to over 17 percent. This is not the whole story, however. The population of pensionable age itself has become older. In 1951, just over one half of them were under the age of 70. By 1976 this proportion had fallen to just under 47 percent. There had been a corresponding increase in the number and proportion of the very old (defined here as meaning the population aged 85 and over). This section of the population makes particularly heavy demands on the medical and social services, and numbers in this group have risen by 133 percent during the last 25 years, from 221 thousand in 1951 to 516 thousand in 1976. During the same period the number of people aged 75–84 has risen from 1.5 million to 2.3 million, an increase of nearly 50 percent. This rise has been brought about partly through the fall in mortality, but mainly because those aged 75–84 in 1976 (that is those born before 1901) are the survivors of larger birth cohorts than was the case for the preceding generations.

The changing sex structure of the population referred to in the Netherlands report is also apparent in Great Britain, where between 1951 and 1976 the age at which the number of women first exceeds the number of men increased from 18 to 45 years. As a consequence, there are now roughly 5% more men than women at the peak marriage ages (20–24 years). During the same period there has been a noticeable decline in the proportion of single males and females. In 1951 roughly a quarter of women aged 15 and over in Great Britain had never been married; by 1976 this proportion had fallen to one fifth. There has also been an increase in the proportion of divorced people, although this trend has been partially offset in recent years by increased remarriage rates among the divorced. It is worth noting that there has been a considerable increase in the proportion of single-person households in Great Britain (from 4% of private households in 1951 to 8% in 1976). Much of this increase can be accounted for by a rise in the number of pensioners living alone.

Given the disparity in cultural traditions and economic development between the North African countries and those in Europe, the focus of demographic concern can be expected to vary accordingly. This is illustrated by the considerable attention given in both the Algerian and Moroccan reports to trends in literacy. In both countries the proportion of the population who are illiterate has fallen over the last 20 years. The improvement for rural women has, however, been marginal. In Morocco, where the illiterate proportion among the total adult population fell from 87% to 75% between 1960 and 1971, the situation for rural women has remained unchanged, 98–99% still being unable to read or write. There is evidence, however, that illiteracy among younger women is declining. According to the Algerian report, in 1977 almost all women aged 50–54 were illiterate, compared with about 60% of those aged 18–20. Even so, girls in rural areas still have the lowest school enrolment, just over 40% attending school in 1977; the corresponding figure for girls in urban areas was 85%.

As a result of high fertility in these countries the population is comparatively "young", with only 5–6% aged 60 and over. Another factor exerting an impact on population composition is the migration of males of working age to other countries in the Region. This movement is examined in greater detail later in this chapter. For the moment it is sufficient to note that until quite recently there were more females than males aged 20–44. This was not (as in the more developed countries) because of higher male mortality but reflects male labour migration.[a] Finally, attention should be drawn to the rapid urbanization taking place in these countries. Morocco's urban population has expanded from 38% to 42% of the total since 1975. In Algeria, where the level of urbanization is similar, the proportion of the population living in urban areas has more than tripled over the last 20 years. Clearly, such changes in population distribution will have major implications for the provision of health and social services, especially since migration to urban centres more often than not implies the effective severance of rural cultural and economic support.

To sum up, declining fertility rates aided by increased survival have brought about a rapid aging of the population in the European Region. This was especially so during the 1960s. Significant changes in the sex structure of the population have occurred in some countries because of the pattern of male migration. In particular, the age at which the excess of males is reversed has risen. It now occurs well into adulthood and not, as in the past, in adolescence. Industrialization and the decline of rural labour have brought about marked changes in population distribution, characterized by a trend towards increasing urbanization.

Family formation

Changing patterns of family formation and dissolution are likely to affect other demographic behaviour in many ways. Thus, to the extent that childbearing largely occurs within marriage, a falling marriage rate, a higher mean age at marriage and an increase in marital disruption are factors that themselves can lead to lower completed fertility rates. Furthermore, marital status has repeatedly been found to be closely related to the propensity to migrate, and it also appears to exert some impact on individual morbidity and survival chances.[b] Consequently, the pattern of family formation is an important aspect of population development with wide-ranging socioeconomic and health implications. Some of the major changes in terms of family formation that have taken place in the European Region of WHO are outlined in Chapter 2. This section will attempt to elaborate further on these

---

[a] As stated in the Moroccan report, this may in part be artefactual because of a greater tendency among women to report a lower than true age.

[b] Whilst the age–marital status relationship to migration has been repeatedly confirmed, with the young and single showing the highest propensity to move, the relationship of marital status to survival is in general less clear. A number of studies have found lower mortality among the married (for males at least) although this in part may reflect differential selection, with those whose health is impaired being less likely to marry.

trends, and focus in greater detail on the recent developments in marriage, divorce, family composition and household size in specific countries.

Changes in marital status

To obtain an overview of the patterns in family formation that have emerged, it is useful first to compare some of the changes in marital status which have taken place in the period 1960–1980. A common development in the Nordic countries, and in fact in most of Northern and Western Europe, has been a decline in the proportion of currently married people and a consistent upward trend in divorce. Data for the Nordic countries reveal that the average annual number of marriages has progressively declined since 1970. By 1979 the total figure had fallen by some 28% in Finland and by 20% in Norway. The number of marriages celebrated each year will, of course, be affected by the age structure of the population, as well as by previous marital patterns. From an analytical perspective, a better alternative is to examine changes in the general marriage rate.[a] In both the Netherlands and Great Britain, marriage rates reached a maximum in 1970 but declined sharply for both sexes thereafter. Interestingly, the data for Great Britain indicate that the decline in marriage was entirely caused by a lower incidence of first marriages, since remarriage rates, in contrast, have risen since 1970. In Belgium the same sort of pattern can be observed, with a large fall in first marriages since the early 1970s. This has been somewhat counterbalanced by an increase in the number of remarriages. During the 1970s there was a consistent increase in the number who went on to marry a second time, with the result that the Belgian remarriage rate increased by about 22% by 1978.

Concurrent with these developments, the frequency of divorce shows a marked upward trend in most European countries. In Great Britain in 1976, for example, there were 10 divorces per 1000 persons married. This is five times the level for the 1956–1960 period. Similarly, whereas 5% of marriages in Sweden in 1976 were dissolved within six years, the corresponding figure for the 1971 marriage cohort was 13%. Data presented in the Norwegian study indicate that for each 10 marriages that took place during the first half of the 1960s one, on average, would end in divorce; in 1980 the comparable number of divorces had risen to three. It is also of interest to note that in several of these countries there are now fewer marriages contracted each year than are dissolved by divorce or death. This has been the case, for instance, in Norway since 1978.

A question that arises from these trends in marriage and divorce is whether more and more people are choosing to remain single throughout the major part of their adult life. This would not, however, appear to be the case in view of the concomitant sharp rise in remarriage rates in these countries. Moreover, from the data available, it appears that cohabitation without marriage has become increasingly common. Surveys in the Nordic

[a] This rate relates the number of individuals who marry in a given year (numerator) to those who are eligible to marry during this period (denominator).

countries indicate that the majority of couples who now marry have previously lived together as a first stage. Information on this trend is relatively scarce in the Netherlands, but an impression can be gained from the number of unmarried persons having "a permanent relationship with the head of the household in which they live". Between 1977 and 1979 this figure increased from 81 000 to 108 000, representing close to 3% of all households of two or more persons. A recent survey of Flemish adolescents underlines the increasing popularity of consensual union in Belgium. According to the survey, close to 50% intended to cohabit with their prospective partners before marriage.

In general, these changes in marriage patterns and the decreasing propensity to marry have been less pronounced in the Eastern European countries. In Hungary, however, a definite decline in marriage is apparent after 1975, the number of marriages falling from 104 000 in that year to some 80 000 in 1980. This decline is not attributable simply to changes in population composition. This is confirmed by the trend in the general marriage rate which fell by 16 per 1000 for males (from 85 to 69) and 14 per 1000 for females (from 65 to 51) over the same period. Part of this decline can be attributed to a decreasing willingness of widowed and divorced persons to remarry. According to the Hungarian report, a decline in the propensity to remarry can be observed since the 1960s. In Czechoslovakia, too, there is some indication that marriage rates have recently shown a downward trend. The latest available figures (1979) for first marriages indicate rates of 78 per 1000 for males and 110 per 1000 for females, compared with 86 and 118, respectively, in 1975. A declining trend is also evident in remarriage rates which have, since 1975, fallen by 7 per 1000 for men (67 to 60) and 1 per 1000 for women (19 to 18).

On the other hand, the increasing incidence of divorce is as apparent in the Eastern European countries as it is elsewhere. Data from the German Democratic Republic indicate that the crude divorce rate in 1979 was 2½ times higher than in 1960. During roughly the same period, the divorce rate in Hungary increased from 1.7 to 2.6 per 1000 population, and the annual number of divorces increased by some 68%. A similar trend appears to obtain in Czechoslovakia, where marital status statistics indicate that the proportion of divorced persons doubled between 1961 and 1979.

In general, the developments in marriage patterns in Southern Europe have been less homogeneous than in other regions, and indeed trends in some of these countries have been quite the reverse of those experienced elsewhere. This is, for example, the case with Greece and Portugal, where marriage rates have been rising since the 1960s. In Greece, first-marriage rates increased by 15% for males and 26% for females between 1961 and 1971. The Portuguese statistics similarly indicate a 40% rise in the rate of first marriages between 1960 and 1975. Since then, however, marriage rates have consistently declined in Portugal suggesting the onset of a new trend. In both countries the first-marriage rates increased as a result of a fall in the mean age at marriage, which, traditionally has been higher in Southern Europe. As a consequence of changing attitudes towards the remarriage of widows, there has been a considerable rise in the proportions who remarry.

Indeed, in Portugal between 1970 and 1978, male remarriage rates doubled while those for women increased threefold.

Cultural, and more specifically religious, pressures have kept divorce rates in Southern Europe comparatively low. Nonetheless, the evidence suggests that, as elsewhere, divorce has been increasing during the period under review. The data included in the Greek report indicate that the incidence of divorce per 1000 married couples rose from 1.3 in 1961 to 2.0 ten years later. Similarly, overall divorce rates trebled in Portugal during the first half of the 1970s, although the level was still only about 0.33 per 1000 in 1975.

In Moslem countries, marriage is virtually universal and for women, at least, generally occurs at a relatively young age. While there is no indication that the popularity of marriage has been declining in Algeria and Morocco, a significant development has been an increase in the mean age at marriage for women. In Algeria, for example, the mean age increased from 18.3 years in 1966 to 20.9 years in 1977. A major consequence of this change is a substantial decline in the proportion of women who were married and exposed to pregnancy by the age of 17 (from 55% to 24% of all women aged 17 years). In contrast, the available data do not point to any particular change in the divorce pattern for these countries. In Morocco, for example, the proportion of the population who were currently divorced hardly changed between 1960 and 1971. It is also of interest to note the comparatively low sex ratio (32 men per 100 women) among the divorced population in Algeria in 1971.[a] Moreover, in the younger age groups (20–29 years) the imbalance of the sexes was even larger. As noted in the country report, a common reason for divorce in Algeria is infertility. This may well be related to the early age at which many women marry and begin their sexual and reproductive life, and it may, subsequently, impede them from remarrying.

Age-specific marriage rates

Summary indicators, such as those presented above, are useful in so far as they communicate the major trends and intercountry differences in marriage and divorce. An individual's chance of marrying, however, largely depends on his or her age. For a more precise understanding of marital patterns, therefore, one must turn to an analysis of age-specific marriage rates. To facilitate cross-cultural comparisons of marriage, the age-specific rates for a number of countries drawn from the various regions of Europe are shown in Fig. 1 and 2 for men and women, respectively.

Although each of the curves follows approximately the same basic pattern, with marriage rates rising to a peak (usually during the third decade of life) and declining rapidly thereafter, there is nonetheless considerable intercountry variation in the chances of marriage for individuals of the same age. For men the most likely age of first marriage is between 25 and 29 years; the exceptions are Portugal, where the peak occurs five years earlier, and

---

[a] In most European countries, the ratio typically varies between 70 and 80, reflecting differences in the chances of remarriage and the differential mortality of the sexes.

Fig. 1. Age-specific first marriage rates for men in selected countries, latest available year

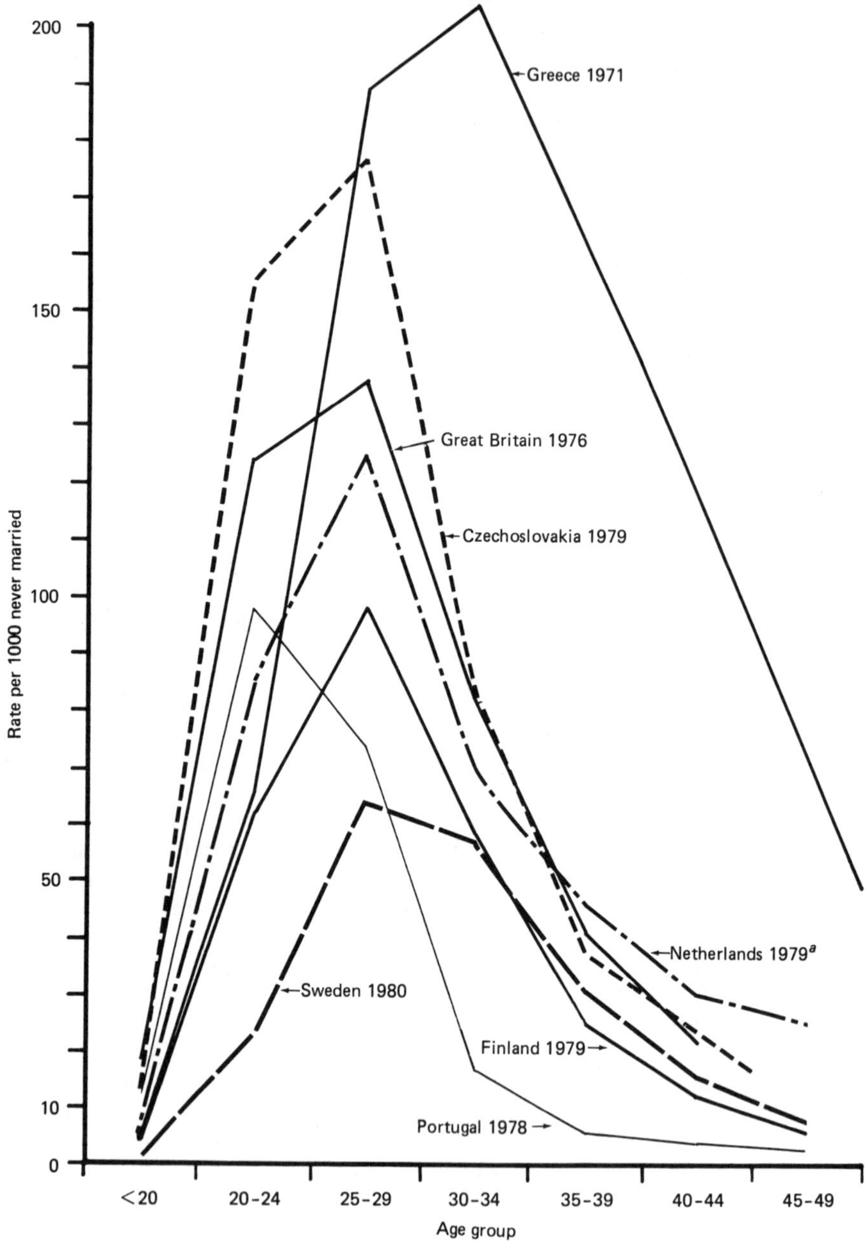

[a] All marriage rates.

Source: Based on data contained in the respective country reports.

Fig. 2. Age-specific first marriage rates for women in selected countries, latest available year

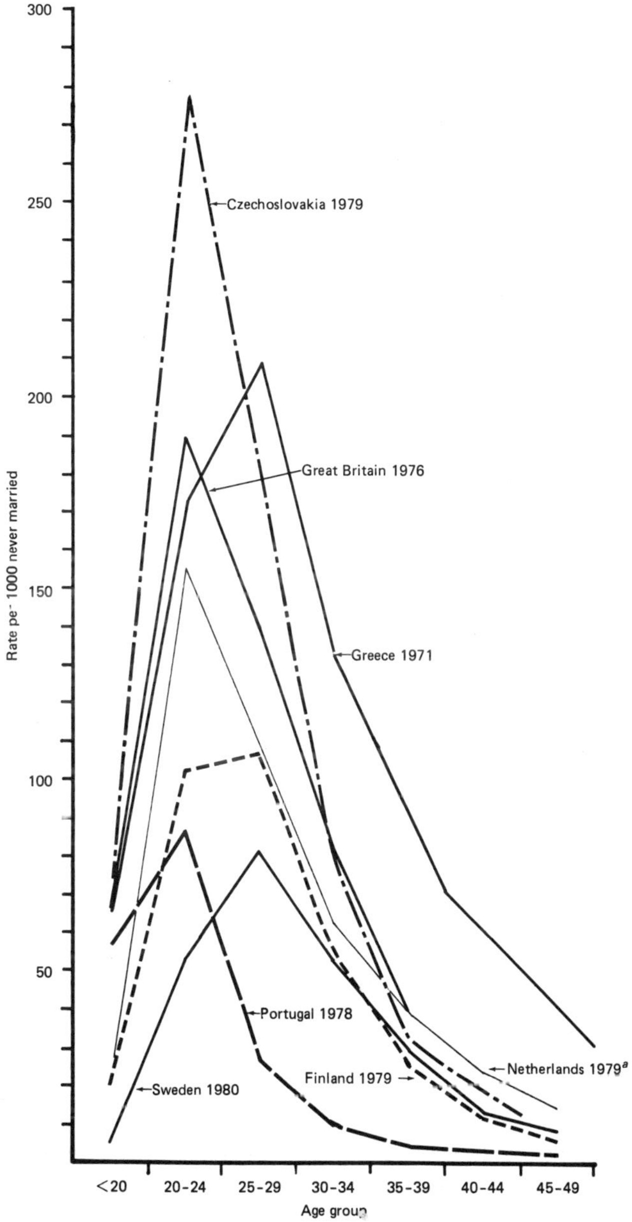

[a] All marriage rates.

Source: Based on data contained in the respective country reports.

Greece where it is delayed to 30–34 years. Moreover, from an inspection of age-specific marriage rates for Greece dating back to 1961, it is clear that this age pattern is not a temporary phenomenon but that it reflects different cultural norms with regard to marriage. In Portugal, on the other hand, a comparison with previous age-specific rates suggests that the current pattern has emerged only since 1975. Before that year the pattern was more typical of the one found in other countries, the maximum likelihood of marriage occurring for those aged 25–29 years. Though less marked, noticeable differences between nations are also evident in the speed with which the chances of contracting a first marriage declines. Thus a single Swedish male who does not marry during the peak ages of 25–29 years has almost the same probability of marrying during the next five years. Conversely, for a Czechoslovakian male of similar age, the chances of marriage are reduced by 50%.

Not surprisingly, perhaps, the female marriage patterns for these same countries show a similar diversity. Compared with males, however, the highest rates for women are generally to be found among those aged 20–24, reflecting the traditional age gap between spouses on first marriage (see Chapter 3). Another interesting difference between the sexes evident from the graphs is that the pattern of female marriage usually displays a sharper peak. In other words, in most countries women marry within a short age span, and a woman who is still single by the age of 30 clearly has much less chance of finding a suitable partner than her male counterpart. What is also remarkable are the substantial intercountry variations in the age pattern of declines in first marriage rates. These undoubtedly reflect the fact that mean age at first marriage began rising in some countries in the 1970s whilst in others the opposite trend occurred. The increase in mean age at marriage has been particularly rapid in the Nordic countries, and this is almost certainly attributable to the pattern of cohabitation leading to a postponement of legal marriage. In Finland and Sweden the average age at first marriage began to increase in the late 1960s and, according to the latest Swedish figures (1980), it is currently 29.0 for men and 26.4 for women. This is all the more impressive when one observes that this represents an increase of 2.8 years for men and 2.4 years for women since 1970. Since the early 1970s a similar trend can also be seen in Great Britain, Luxembourg and the Netherlands and, to a lesser extent, in Czechoslovakia and Hungary.

Concurrent with this increase in age at first marriage, there has been a noticeable decrease in the average age at remarriage in some countries. The data for Czechoslovakia, Finland, Greece, the Netherlands and Norway all reveal a tendency towards a younger age at remarriage during the 1970s. Furthermore, whenever the data permit a distinction to be made between the widowed and the divorced populations, it appears that this trend is either entirely or predominantly the result of earlier remarriage among the divorced. As suggested in the Norwegian report, the reduction in age at remarriage is undoubtedly a consequence of the rapid rise in the size of the divorced population, particularly at younger ages. One should also note the considerable sex differential in the propensity to remarry. Indeed, it is not uncommon for the male rate to be 2–3 times higher than that for women. Part of this imbalance is admittedly a function of differences in the age structure of men and women at risk. Nonetheless, from a comparison of age-specific rates it is clear that the sex differential in remarriage is already apparent at the age of 25 years. Moreover, there is no evidence to suggest that the gap between the sexes with regard to remarriage is decreasing.

Age-specific divorce rates

Even though the frequency of divorce differs widely among countries in the European Region, a comparison of rates prevailing around 1960 and 1980 indicates that, irrespective of the initial level, marital dissolutions were typically 2–3 times more frequent at the end of the period. As is clear from Fig. 3, which shows the age pattern of divorce for women in selected countries, the frequency of divorce is also closely related to age. Although not shown, the pattern for males is similar, the principal difference being that the peak in rates occurs five years later for men. The fact that the highest divorce rates coincide with the ages at which marriage is also at its peak tends to suggest that most couples who divorce do so relatively soon after getting married. For most of the countries included in the graph, more than half the divorces were from marriages that had lasted less than ten years. In general, the data suggest that the fourth and fifth years of marriage constitute the period of highest risk. This would account for the comparatively low rates among persons under 20 years of age in most countries. Moreover, from a cohort analysis of divorce, it would appear that adolescent brides have the highest probability of divorce. In Great Britain, for example, of those who married before the age of 20 in 1951, one fifth were divorced by 1976, compared with only 11% for all women who married before the age of 45 in that same year.

As was observed for marriage, the speed with which divorce rates decline from their peak level varies somewhat from country to country. Among the Scandinavian countries, for example, the divorce rate for women aged 40–44 years is still about half of the maximum level, while in Czechoslovakia and the German Democratic Republic the fall is much more rapid, with the rates being closer to one third of that found for women aged 20–24 years. It is also clear from Fig. 3 that variations in the overall level of divorce among countries arise mainly because of the differences at younger ages. Indeed, with the exception of Sweden and Portugal, where legislation and cultural norms have kept divorce rates exceptionally low at all ages, the variations in rates among the other countries above age 40 are comparatively minor.

It is interesting to ask whether the general increase in divorce since the 1960s has resulted from a secular trend affecting all age groups or, rather, from changes in behaviour at certain ages. Judging from the age-specific data included in the country reports, it appears that all age groups have contributed to the rise. In most cases, however, the age contributions have not been uniform. In Hungary, divorce rates increased much faster among the very young (under 20 years of age), among women in their thirties and among males aged 35–39 years. A similar pattern, with particularly large increases for those under 20 years of age, can be observed in Czechoslovakia. In 1979 the divorce rate for men in this age group had increased by

Fig. 3. Age-specific divorce rates for married women in selected countries, latest available year

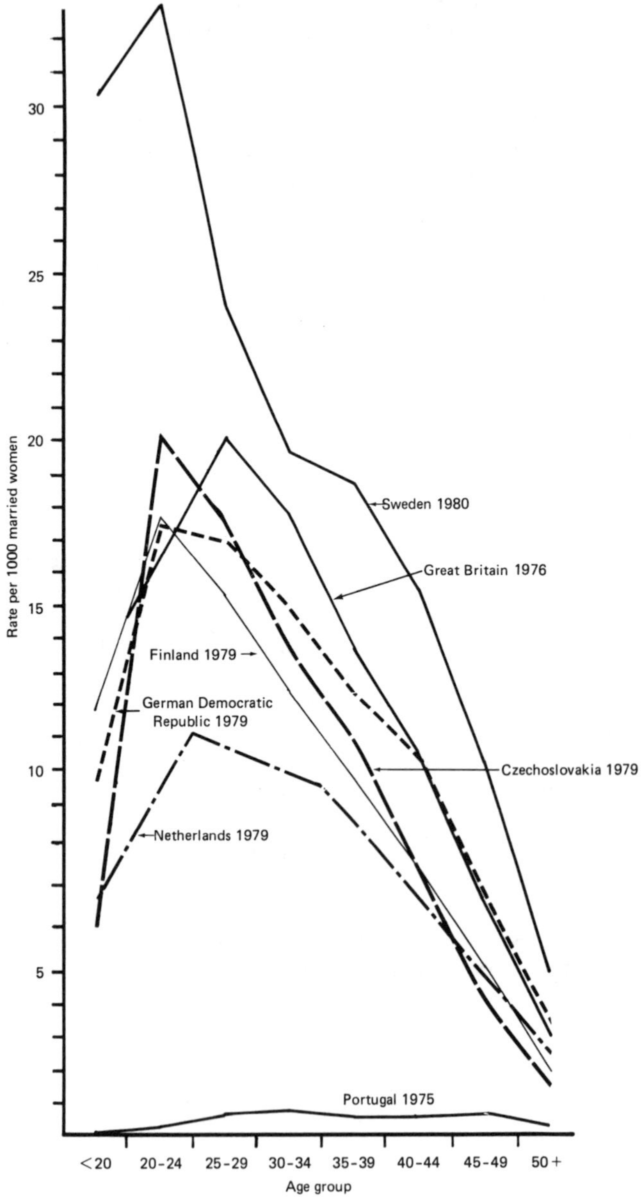

Notes: Great Britain <25 years.
Netherlands 20-29, 30-39, 40-49 year age groups; rates include judicial separations.

Source: Based on data presented in the respective country reports.

a factor of 2.9 compared with the 1960 figure, and for women the increase was almost as large (2.5 times). In the German Democratic Republic, on the other hand, the rise appears to have been roughly uniform in all age groups under 40 years of age. A comparison of the 1965 and 1976 divorce frequencies for Great Britain indicates a disproportionate increase among persons under 25 years of age and also among the older middle aged. As noted in the British report, the increase in the divorce rate of this latter group is probably related to changes in divorce legislation which, since 1971, has made it easier for couples whose marriage has terminated *de facto* to obtain a divorce.

Over the last 20 years, marital dissolutions have tripled in the Netherlands. Divorce rates appear to have increased at roughly the same pace in all age groups, with the exception of a slower rate for those under 20 years. This apparent uniformity, however, could in part reflect the fact that Dutch divorce statistics are tabulated in 10-year age groups. Conversely, in Finland and Norway the growth in divorce has been particularly rapid among men aged between 30 and 44 years and for women in their thirties. Although divorce rates for these age groups have also risen rapidly in Sweden, the trend is overshadowed by the spectacular rise in divorce among the very young: between 1973 and 1980 the age-specific divorce rate of women under 20 years of age soared from 4.2 to 30.3 per 1000 married.

Unfortunately, data limitations preclude a comparable analysis of marital dissolution in the North African countries of the Region. Nonetheless, judging from the proportion of the population who were divorced in Algeria and Morocco in 1970, the frequency of divorce would seem to be comparable to, and indeed may even exceed, that of many Western European countries.[a] Moreover, since the likelihood of remarriage for men is much higher in Moslem societies, females typically constitute a much larger share of the divorced population. In Algeria, for instance, 3.8% of adult females in 1971 were divorced — more than three times the proportion for males (1.2%).

Trends in average household size

Changes in marital frequency and in the average age at marriage, the growing acceptance of other forms of cohabitation, and the increasing propensity for marriage to end in divorce all have implications for family formation and composition. Moreover, changes in family norms and in the role of women, together with the widespread use of contraception, have severely reduced average family size in most countries. Commenting on some of these developments, the Swedish report notes that since 1960 there has been a marked increase in the proportion of single-person households (from 20% to 30%) and a corresponding decline in those with five or more persons (from 13% to 7%). At the same time, the proportion of single-parent

[a] By way of comparison, the divorced population in Morocco in 1970 constituted 1.6% of the total, whereas in the Netherlands in 1969 this group accounted for less than 1%. Indeed, given the younger age structure of the Moroccan population, the difference would have appeared even larger had it been possible to base the comparison on adults only.

families and families with children born to other parents has grown considerably. Indeed, a recent survey (1980) in Sweden reported that one in ten of the children covered by the study lived in single-parent families, and about the same proportion lived in "mixed" families as described above. A similar trend can also be observed outside Scandinavia, particularly in the Western European region.

Later in Chapter 2 the distinct drop in average household size is shown to be largely attributable to fewer large families (with five or more members) and more consisting of just a single person. In some countries, however, the proportion of households with two members has also increased quite markedly. This is the case, for instance, in the Netherlands, where household composition statistics indicate that households consisting of a married couple only increased from 20% in 1960 to 25% in 1977/78. According to the Dutch report, the reasons for this trend probably lie in the increasing popularity of deliberate childlessness, the postponement of births among the newly married, and the younger average age at which children leave home.

The sharp rise in single-person households is largely a function of the increasing longevity of the elderly, coupled with an apparently greater unwillingness of children to take a surviving parent into their home. Data from the Belgian report indicate that among the very old (80 years and over) 23% of men and 37% of women were living alone in 1976. Similarly, in Luxembourg men constitute less than a third of the single-person households. This pattern is repeated in many other countries as well, and arises because of the differential mortality between the sexes at earlier stages of life, especially during later middle age. Another significant feature suggested by the Luxembourg report is that the overwhelming majority (63%) of females living alone in 1979 were widows. To the extent that family support systems for these women remain functional, their health and social care needs will differ from those who had never been married (9%). These considerations must also be borne in mind for men living alone, roughly half (46%) of whom, in Luxembourg at least, were single.

The tendency towards a reduction in average household size has been much less evident in Eastern Europe. In fact, it is only in Hungary that mean household size has actually declined. Furthermore, the changes in household and family composition that occurred in Hungary are much the same as those that occurred elsewhere. Thus, the share of single-person households increased from 15% in 1960 to almost 20% in 1980. Over the same period, the proportion of families consisting of a couple only increased from 31% to 35%. Families with four or more children decreased from 5.1% to 1.7% of the total. These trends, moreover, are not exclusively caused by changes in fertility and in the living arrangements of children. As the Hungarian report suggests, the growth of the family type "couple without children" has in part arisen as a result of increased life expectancy.

Contrary to the experience of most other countries, the mean number of persons per household has increased in the German Democratic Republic mainly because of a reduction in the number of households with one or two members and an increase in those with four, five and particularly six persons living together. The rise in single-person households in Czechoslovakia, on the other hand, was countered by other modifications in household composition, the net result being that average household size remained essentially unchanged.

Despite the considerable reduction in average household size that has occurred in most countries of Southern Europe, the highest mean family size is still to be found there. The decline in fertility began later in these countries and family ties have remained comparatively strong. Nonetheless, many of the compositional changes in household structure have been in accord with those experienced elsewhere in Europe. Thus, in the 1960s the share of single- and two-person households increased in Greece and Portugal while, in relative terms, those with five or more members declined. In fact, households of this latter type (which in both countries accounted for some 32% of all private dwellings in the early 1960s) had declined to 22% and 27%, respectively, in Greece and Portugal by the end of the decade. Changing socioeconomic conditions and lower fertility have undoubtedly been the main factors underlying this decline, aided by increased internal and international migration.

As one might expect, household compositional changes in Algeria between 1966 and 1977 differed in a number of respects from the pattern observed in other countries of the European Region. During that time, the average number of persons per household rose from 5.9 to 6.7. Underlying this change are two distinct trends. On the one hand, there has been a noticeable increase in the proportion of households containing eight or more persons (from 27% to 37%). On the other hand, the share of households with five or less members has declined. A major factor contributing to these developments is the reduction in mortality, particularly among infants and young children. However, as suggested in the Algerian report, part of the increase in average household size may well have resulted from the increasing shortage of housing; in 1977, for example, the mean number of persons per room was no less than 3.5.

Implications for women

The changes in family formation and dissolution discussed in this section have had important implications for the economic role of women. As a consequence of small family norms, most women in the industrialized countries of the Region have completed their childbearing by their early thirties and are then ready to re-enter the workforce. Another factor that has contributed to the increase in working women is the rise in the number of marriages ending in divorce, and the tendency for couples to divorce at earlier ages. The widespread implications of this development are not discussed in the country reports, although the significance of the trend can be gauged from the information provided on the employment status of family members. In 1960 in Sweden, for example, cases where both husband and wife worked outside the home accounted for only about one fifth of all families, with two thirds of couples following the traditional pattern of the man only being economically active. Fifteen years later, however, the proportions had altered to 50% and 27%, respectively. A similar development has occurred in Finland where, according to the country report, the proportion of married couples with only the husband working fell sharply from 45% to 26% between 1970 and 1975. In Hungary also, households with two breadwinners have become relatively more common, increasing from 48% in 1970 to 53% in 1980. At the same time, however, because of the aging of populations, several countries have witnessed a noticeable rise in the proportion of households with only inactive members. This has been the case in Hungary, where the proportion of such households has increased from 16% to 23% over the last decade.

By way of summary, a few general observations on trends in family formation in the European Region may be made here. Given the wide variation in national customs and attitudes that affect such behaviour. the diversity of country trends is not surprising. In this context, however, it is interesting to note the virtually universal tendency towards a decline in the number of marriages celebrated and an increase in divorce. Accompanying these changes, there has been a noticeable increase in cohabitation outside of marriage in many countries, leading to a rise in the mean age of first marriage. Average family size has also decreased, as has average household size, although the reduction is less evident in Eastern Europe. In particular, there has been a marked increase in the number of single-person households, many of them consisting of elderly people. In some countries, the number of two-person households has also risen.

Fertility and family planning

With the completion of the mortality transition in the greater part of the European Region, fertility has long been the most important determinant of population growth. The history of European fertility is described in Chapter 3. Despite the fact that birth rates in many European countries have fallen to unprecedently low levels, the current pattern of fertility and developments in the 1960–1980 period have varied substantially in the Region. This is reflected in the total fertility rates (TFRs) shown in Table 3.[a]

Between 1960 and 1970 most countries experienced a decline in overall fertility as measured by TFR. The reduction was particularly marked in Finland, the Netherlands and Norway. In other populations, where the level of fertility was lower at the start of the period, the declines were more modest. In Portugal, however, fertility began to fall substantially only after 1970. The rates in most of the countries shown in Table 3 continued to decline throughout the next decade with only minor fluctuations. The notable exceptions to this pattern were Czechoslovakia, where fertility actually increased, and Greece and Hungary, where the levels at the end of the 1970s were similar to those prevailing 20 or so years earlier.

As a consequence of the gradual decline of both birth and death rates, net reproduction rates (NRRs) in most of the countries shown in Table 3 had

[a] The TFR is a summary indicator of the prevailing level of fertility, calculated as the sum of age-specific fertility rates.

Table 3. Development of total fertility rates between 1960 and 1980 in selected countries in the WHO European Region

Country	Total fertility rate in:			
	1960	1970	latest available year	
Algeria	—	7.86	7.36	(1977)
Belgium	2.58	2.20	1.73	(1976)
Czechoslovakia	2.39	2.07	2.33	(1979)
Finland	2.71	1.83	1.64	(1979)
German Democratic Republic	2.33	2.19	1.89	(1979)
Great Britain	2.69	2.44	1.70	(1977)
Greece	2.28	2.34	2.26	(1978)
Hungary	2.02	1.97	1.92	(1980)
Luxembourg	2.28	1.97	1.46	(1978)
Morocco	—	7.60[a]	—	
Netherlands	3.12	2.57	1.57	(1979)
Norway	2.94[b]	2.24[c]	1.72	(1980)
Portugal	3.13	3.11	2.11	(1978)
Sweden	2.17	1.94	1.68	(1980)

[a] CERED estimate, which refers only to the north-western part of the country.

[b] Period 1961–1965.

[c] Period 1971–1975.

Source: Country reports.

already dropped below replacement by the mid 1970s. Indeed, in Greece and Hungary this occurred as early as 1960. According to the Hungarian report, various social measures were taken in the second half of the 1960s to encourage women to have more children, with the result that the NRR temporarily rose (1974–1977) above replacement. In Greece, where no special incentives appear to have been introduced, the NRR increased spontaneously from a comparatively low level of 0.976 in 1960 to 1.074 in 1975. As noted in the Greek report, both higher fertility and declines in mortality contributed to this development. An NRR below unity was also evident in Czechoslovakia, Finland, Luxembourg and Sweden prior to 1970. In Czechoslovakia, however, fertility incentives and restrictions on the availability of abortion contributed to a subsequent rise in the NRR to 1.184 by 1974; since then the rate has progressively fallen.

Age-specific fertility rates

A major limitation of any summary index of fertility is that it does not, of course, provide any insight into the actual pattern of childbearing. This may vary considerably from one population to another, depending on marriage habits, the use of family planning methods, and other factors. That this is the case can be seen from Table 4, which gives age-specific fertility rates for the various countries in the Region. Although these rates display the same general shape and trend, there are nonetheless a number of interesting variations. The fertility schedules can be classified according to three basic types: those with an early peak, those where the peak occurs later in the childbearing period, and those with a relatively broad peak characterized by approximately constant fertility over two contiguous age groups. The majority of countries included in Table 4 demonstrate the late peak pattern, with fertility reaching a maximum in the age group 25–29. In Czechoslovakia, the German Democratic Republic and Hungary, however, age-specific fertility during both decades, 1960–1970 and 1970–1980, was highest for women aged 20–24 years. Interestingly, in some countries a transition in the age pattern of fertility occurred during the period under consideration. In Finland and Norway the peak shifted to the later ages while the opposite trend was observed in Greece and Portugal.

A characteristic of declining fertility is that childbearing tends to become increasingly concentrated in a relatively narrow segment of the reproductive lifespan. This can be seen clearly from Table 4. It is also evident that the largest relative declines have occurred among women aged 30 years and under. Almost certainly, older women reduced their fertility in the 1960s and early 1970s because they had achieved their desired family size (see, for example, the Norwegian report). Another interesting feature suggested by Table 4 is the existence of contrasting trends in fertility among the youngest women. In the Scandinavian countries, as well as in Luxembourg and the Netherlands, births to women aged under 20 have decreased markedly, whereas the opposite trend is apparent in the countries of Southern and Eastern Europe.

Given that the risk of complications of pregnancy and childbirth is greatest among adolescents and older women, the age structure of fertility has important implications for both maternal and infant health. In 1960 about one fifth of all births occurring in this latter group of countries were to women in the least favourable age groups — i.e. under 20 and above 35 years of age. By 1980 the dispersion of births had, in most cases, contracted. In Algeria and Morocco, however, about one third of all children are born to mothers in these age groups; and in Greece, Hungary and Portugal the proportion is still about one fifth. In these last three countries, though, there has been a substantial reduction in the relative number of births occurring to women over 35 years of age which has been accompanied by a concomitant rise in adolescent fertility.

Family planning and abortion

Apart from the cultural values that influence family size and composition, differences in fertility levels and patterns in Europe are closely related to the use of contraception and abortion. An overview of intercountry variation in the European Region in the use of family planning and in the practice of abortion can be found in Chapter 3 of this book. In this section, therefore, attention will be restricted to specific information contained in the country reports.

In view of the comparatively high fertility levels prevailing in Algeria and Morocco, it is not surprising to find that birth control in these countries is practised by only a small proportion of couples. According to the data furnished by Morocco, new family planning acceptors in 1980 constituted less than 3% of women of reproductive age. As the report suggests, this is insignificant given the high discontinuation rates. At the other extreme are countries such as those in Scandinavia, where contraceptive knowledge and use are extremely widespread even among the very young. Interestingly, an increasing proportion of couples are opting for sterilization once the desired number of children has been achieved. Further, in these same countries, liberal abortion laws reduce the number of unwanted pregnancies.

Not only does the use of modern methods of birth control vary markedly among countries in the Region, but also the choice of contraceptive method appears to be very much a function of the woman's age. In all the countries for which information is available, the use of oral contraception appears to be consistently higher among younger women. In 1977 in Norway, for example, some 30% of women under the age of 25 years used oral contraceptives. The popularity of this method declined extremely rapidly beyond this age. A survey carried out around the same time among the Flemish community in Belgium found that about 60% of contraceptive users under age 25 used the Pill. Although the proportion using this method also fell monotonically with increasing age, the decline was much less rapid than in Norway. For example, only 9% of Norwegian women over 40 years of age were using oral contraceptives; in Belgium the proportion was one fifth. The pattern in the Netherlands around 1980 closely resembled that in Belgium, with a high proportion of women taking the Pill, including women in their forties. In the Netherlands, however, recent data (for the period 1975–1979) point to a noticeable decline in the use of oral contraceptives among women aged 30–39 years. In Hungary, on the other hand, the overall use of oral contraception has increased particularly rapidly, so that in 1977 almost half of all women who reported using a birth control method were taking the Pill. Even among women in their late thirties, the proportion using oral contraceptives was close to one third.

Although some differential age patterns are also evident for other contraceptive methods, they do not appear to be as pronounced or as consistent as those found for oral contraception. Thus, for instance, the use of the condom hardly varies by age in Finland, Norway and the Flemish part of Belgium, whereas Dutch and Hungarian couples increasingly rely on this method with advancing age. The use of the IUD, on the other hand, is usually most common among women aged 25–34 years.

In those European countries where abortion is freely available, it would appear that its main effect has been to reduce extramarital fertility and births to older married women. For example, the British report estimates

Table 4. Age-specific fertility rates for selected countries, 1960–1980

Country	Year	Age group (in years)						
		15–19	20–24	25–29	30–34	35–39	40–44	45–49
Algeria	1970	132.4	347.6	363.6	330.3	258.1	122.3	17.0
	1977	97.0	284.6	341.6	336.3	266.8	128.7	17.3
Belgium	1960	24.9	150.1	162.3	99.1	50.4	16.8	1.1
	1976	26.8	118.4	121.6	55.0	19.0	4.6	0.4
Czechoslovakia	1960	46.0[a]	198.7	131.7	63.8	29.1	8.8	0.6
	1979	53.6[a]	210.8	127.5	53.2	17.2	3.0	0.2
Finland	1960	29.3[a]	163.5	158.7	103.9	61.3	25.0	—
	1979	19.3[a]	93.1	113.1	68.3	27.5	6.4	0.3
German Democratic Republic	1960	65.0	168.9	125.7	67.4	31.1	7.5	—
	1979	67.9	175.7	94.0	31.2	8.5	1.5	—
Great Britain	1960[b]	34.0	165.6	171.9	100.8	46.4	13.8	0.8
	1976	33.0	111.0	120.0	58.0	19.0	4.0	—
Greece	1960	17.4[a]	109.7	157.5	105.7	48.6	14.4	2.0
	1978	50.0[a]	158.3	135.8	71.3	28.9	7.1	0.8
Hungary	1960	52.5	159.2	105.6	52.9	25.0	3.6[c]	
	1980	68.0	158.6	100.0	40.9	13.7	1.5	
Luxembourg	1960	23.2	142.9	149.5	90.4	37.9	11.9	1.0
	1978	17.1	91.4	106.4	53.7	20.0	3.6	0.3

Table 4 (contd)

Morocco	1972	74.0	326.9	378.5	321.9	233.4	155.8	30.1
Netherlands	1960	17.0	121.7	208.0	152.4	88.5	33.1	2.6
	1979	8.9	82.2	139.2	63.3	16.9	3.2	0.3
Norway	1961–1965	37.9	178.0	177.3	112.7	58.1	18.7	1.3
	1980	25.2	108.3	122.4	62.8	21.9	4.1	0.2
Portugal	1960	26.6[a]	148.9	171.2	127.9	92.5	43.5	3.9
	1979	41.1	138.3	123.5	78.2	36.2	15.2	1.9
Sweden	1960	34.5	128.6	136.7	82.6	38.9	12.2	0.8
	1980	15.8	95.6	124.2	70.7	24.9	4.3	0.2

[a] Includes births to women under 15 years.

[b] England & Wales only.

[c] Women aged 40–49 years.

that in 1976, some 38% of all pregnancies occurring outside marriage were terminated compared with 7% of conceptions within marriage. In the Netherlands, too, the fall in illegitimate births in the mid-1970s has been attributed to the increasing use of abortion and contraception.

An overview of abortion trends in Europe during the 1970s can be found in Chapter 3. What is not apparent from these data, however, is the age structure of women seeking an abortion and whether or not this has altered appreciably in recent years. Fig. 4 illustrates the considerable variation in age-specific abortion rates in some of the countries in the Region. In the Nordic countries, abortion rates reach a peak among women aged 20–24, then decline rapidly for women in their late twenties and at a somewhat slower rate for women in their thirties. Thereafter, a sharp decline is again evident, commencing somewhat later in Finland. In the Eastern European countries the peak of the age curve is much more pronounced, and it occurs at a later age. In Hungary, for example, the highest abortion rates are found among women in their early thirties. A contrast to both these patterns is found in the Netherlands. Here, there is relatively little variation with age up to about the age of 40; after this age abortion rates decline quite rapidly.

According to the data from Czechoslovakia, neither the level nor the age pattern of abortion has changed markedly since 1960. For Hungary, on the other hand, the sharp fall in the overall abortion rate appears to have been accompanied by a shift towards the older ages; prior to 1970 abortion rates for women aged 20–24 were consistently higher than those for women in their thirties. In Sweden, the current age pattern is a reflection of the progressive liberalization of the abortion laws. During the 1960s the age curve resembled that for the Netherlands (see Fig. 4), i.e. the rates were roughly uniform for all age groups up to 40. A somewhat similar situation prevailed in Finland until 1970. The markedly higher rates for women under 25 years of age became apparent only after that date, with the introduction of more liberal abortion laws.

The ages at which abortion has the greatest relative impact on fertility rates varies among countries according to the country-specific abortion and fertility schedules. In the Netherlands and in Scandinavia, for example, the largest relative reduction in fertility occurs among the youngest and the oldest women. In the Nordic countries, in fact, abortion rates among women under 20 years of age and over the age of 40 years usually exceed fertility rates. In Eastern Europe, on the other hand, the effect on fertility is greatest for women over 30 years of age.

An interesting trend in contraceptive behaviour is apparent in a number of European countries; this is the more frequent use of irreversible methods. Unfortunately, comparisons are frequently hindered by the general lack of information about the annual number of sterilizations performed. Moreover, some gynaecological operations carried out for therapeutic indications may have a sterilizing effect. In the Netherlands, the annual vasectomy rate has trebled since 1972, and the rate of female sterilization has more than doubled. As might be expected, the operation is most common for both men and women at ages 35–44 years, i.e. after the desired family size has been achieved. A survey in Great Britain in 1975 found that in 25% of

Fig. 4. Age-specific abortion rates in selected European countries, 1979–1980

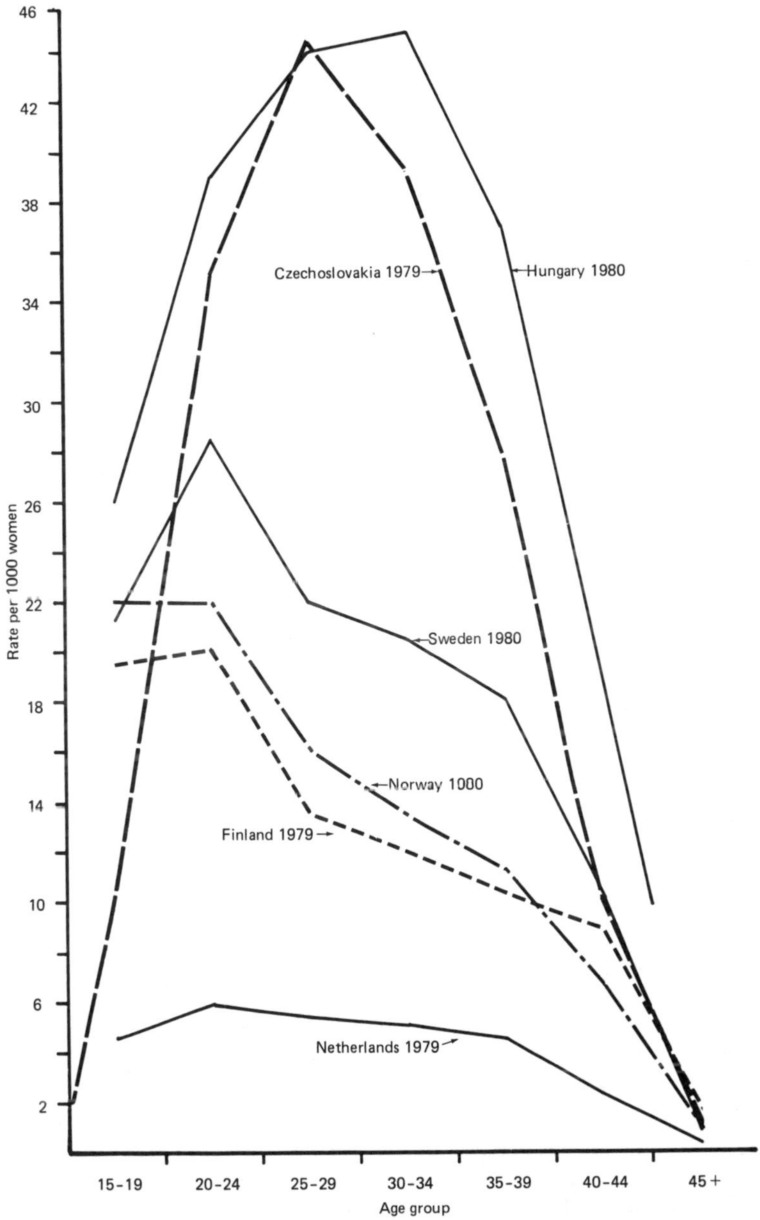

Source: Based on data contained in the respective country reports.

couples aged 35–39 one or other partner had been sterilized. A similar parity-specific relationship can be identified with the rate of sterilization increasing sharply after the birth of the second child. It is also interesting to note that in Sweden the annual number of sterilizations increased fivefold from 1863 in 1970 to 10 202 in 1980. The increase is particularly impressive for men; their share of sterilizations increased from 0.3% of the total in 1970 to 33% just ten years later.

Fertility differentials in Europe

Finally, a number of country reports presented information on socioeconomic and other differentials in fertility within national populations. The existence of differentials between population subgroups in reproductive behaviour has, of course, important implications for the projection of trends in overall fertility. Moreover, with changing social and economic conditions, reproductive behaviour may alter and this, too, can have health and sociodemographic consequences. In some countries, notably Algeria, Greece and Morocco, substantial differences between the fertility of urban and rural women are evident. In 1972 the TFR for urban women in Morocco was 6.6, compared with a rate of 7.8 for those living in rural areas. However, as the Algerian report notes, much of the demographic impact of the fertility differential between the two population groups is effectively eliminated by the difference in mortality.

As a consequence of urbanization, with mainly younger people migrating to the cities, the urban–rural differential in fertility has generally diminished. This is very evident from the Finnish and Greek studies. However, it is important to recognize that socioeconomic differences often underlie urban–rural and other regional variations in fertility. Thus, the higher average number of children per family reported for the non-urban areas of Norway is, in large part, a reflection of the concentration of farmers and fishermen in these areas. In Norway at least, those belonging to these occupational groups have an average of one more child than, for instance, clerical and other "white collar" workers. A similar disparity between major occupation groups is also apparent for Hungary; average completed family size in 1980 was 2.4 children for workers in agriculture, 2.1 for those in non-agricultural manual occupations, and 1.6 for non-manual workers. As suggested in the Hungarian report, a reduction in the agricultural workforce will almost certainly lead to a further decline in Hungarian fertility.

In Great Britain, average completed family size based on 1971 data appears to follow a U-shaped distribution according to social class. Skilled non-manual workers had the lowest mean number of children (2.02) and professional people slightly more (2.06), the highest number of children per family (2.74) being found among unskilled workers. These "aggregate" differentials in fertility reflect, of course, the net impact of differentials in a variety of deterministic factors including earlier marriage, less awareness (or less efficient use) of family planning, and a greater propensity of some couples to have large families. As the Belgian report notes, in commenting on the increasing rarity of large families among certain social classes, "undesired large families, though decreasing in number, tend to occur among couples characterized by an accumulation of unfavourable social and biological characteristics".

The relationship between education and fertility — which, because of smaller family ideals and more effective fertility control, usually results in lower completed fertility for the more educated — is widely recognized. In Europe, reproductive differentials among families of the lowest and highest educational levels have tended to diminish in recent years although they are, nonetheless, still evident. Thus in 1980, completed fertility among women in Hungary with tertiary education was more than 40% lower than that of women with less than eight years of schooling. In the Netherlands, too, family size was found to decrease monotonically with the educational level of the mother, while the relationship to the father's educational level tended to fit a U-shaped curve.

Several countries reported substantial fertility differentials between local and foreign-born women, the latter usually being more fertile. In Great Britain, for example, the TFR in 1971 was 2.4 for all places of birth combined, but 3.1 for those born outside the United Kingdom. The highest TFR (5.4) was reported for Bangladeshis, Indians and Pakistanis residing in Britain. Indeed, the impact of immigrants from the New Commonwealth countries[a] on the overall fertility level and rate of population growth in Great Britain is far from insignificant. In 1976, for example, this group constituted only about 3% of the total population but accounted for some 7% of all live births occurring during that year. Moreover, as a result of their desire for large families, no less than one fifth of all births of fifth children and above occur to women who had emigrated from these countries.

Similarly, data presented in the Dutch report indicate that the general fertility rate of the foreign population in 1978 was more than double that of indigenous women. This differential was largely a result of the much higher fertility among older foreign women, as well as that of women under 20 years of age. However, as noted by both the British and Dutch studies, it may be expected that with increasing assimilation the fertility differential between immigrants and the host population will diminish.

To summarize, marked declines in fertility are evident for most countries in the Region. These declines have been accompanied by a greater concentration of childbearing within a relatively narrow segment of reproductive life (20–34 years), and this has lessened the risk of health impairment for both mother and child. Contraceptive practice varies widely among countries, with an increasing preference for oral contraception among younger women. Furthermore, differentials in fertility between urban and rural populations, between women with different educational levels, and between immigrant and host populations have persisted despite social and economic modernization.

[a] New Commonwealth countries are understood here to include all Commonwealth countries except Australia, Canada and New Zealand.

Mortality

Of the various demographic phenomena, none has greater relevance for describing the health situation and for guiding the formulation of health and social policy than the study of mortality. However, it must be recognized that for most causes of illness, the incidence and prevalence — principal concerns in public health planning — are often poorly reflected by the underlying mortality rates. In the absence of historical information on morbidity that is both comprehensive and comparable, international comparisons of the changing health situation must necessarily continue to be based on existing mortality records, despite their limitations and pitfalls.

Trends in life expectancy

Probably the most widely used measure of mortality is the expectation of life at birth,[a] which summarizes the current age pattern of mortality in the form of a single index which is independent of population age structure. Trends in this measure over the last 20 or so years for selected countries in the Region are shown in Table 5. A number of characteristic patterns can be observed. In the Scandinavian countries and in the Netherlands, very little progress has been made in extending life expectancy for males. To some extent this reflects the comparatively high levels of life expectancy already enjoyed in these countries by 1960, but it has also occurred as the result of a deterioration in mortality conditions, particularly among middle aged men. In the Netherlands, for example, death rates among males aged 40–80 were rising until the mid-1970s, although since then a noticeable decline has occurred. According to the Norwegian report, a 40-year-old Norwegian male can currently expect to live, on average, only one month longer than his counterpart in 1961–1965 and a full year less than a 40-year-old man around 1951–1955. Much the same pattern can be observed in Sweden. Among women, on the other hand, death rates have continued to fall with the result that the sex difference in mortality has widened dramatically over that period in these countries.[b]

Similarly, in the Eastern European countries there has been comparatively little change over the last decade or so in life expectancy for males. Indeed, in Hungary male life expectancy has actually declined since the mid-1960s, although further gains have been recorded for females. In Czechoslovakia, too, male life expectancy at birth decreased by more than 1½ years during the 1960s. It has subsequently risen again to a level more or less equivalent to that prevailing 20 years ago. Mortality conditions among

---

[a] Life expectancy is actually an index of survival rather than of mortality although the two concepts are, of course, directly related to one another.

[b] Between 1950–1954 and 1975–1978, the gap in life expectancy at birth between the sexes widened by 3.2 years in Denmark, 4.1 years in the Netherlands, 3.0 years in Norway and 3.4 years in Sweden, by far the largest increments in the Region. *See* **Lopez, A.D.** The changing sex differential in mortality in developed countries. *In*: Lopez, A.D. & Ruzicka, L.T., ed. *Sex differences in mortality: trends, determinants and consequences.* Canberra, Australian National University Press, 1983.

Table 5. Trends in life expectancy at birth in selected countries of the European Region, 1960–1980

Country	Life expectancy at birth					
	Males			Females		
	1960	1970	Around 1980[a]	1960	1970	Around 1980[a]
Algeria (North)	—	53.4	54.2	—	53.7	56.1
Belgium	66.3	67.3	69.0	72.2	73.7	75.6
Czechoslovakia	67.8	66.2	67.5	73.2	72.9	74.6
England & Wales	68.2[b]	69.1[c]	70.2	74.2[b]	75.4[c]	76.2
Finland	65.4[b]	66.7[c]	68.9	72.6[b]	75.2[c]	77.2
German Democratic Republic	66.5	68.1	68.7	71.4	73.3	74.8
Greece	67.3	70.1	72.9	70.4	73.6	77.6
Hungary	66.4	66.8	66.0	70.6	72.6	73.2
Luxembourg	66.1	67.0[d]	69.0	71.9	73.9[d]	76.2
Morocco	47.3[e]	51.4[c]	—	49.0[e]	51.6[c]	—
Netherlands	71.1[b]	71.2[c]	72.4	75.9[b]	77.2[c]	78.9
Norway	71.0[b]	71.4[c]	72.3	76.0[b]	77.7[c]	78.7
Portugal	61.6[b]	64.6[c]	67.3	67.3[b]	71.0[c]	74.2
Sweden	71.2	72.2	72.8	74.9	77.1	78.8

[a] Figures shown are for the latest available year.

[b] 1960–1964 or 1961–1965.

[c] 1970–1974 or 1971–1975.

[d] 1971–1973.

[e] 1962–1972.

Source: Respective country reports except for England & Wales, Greece and Portugal (1978) and Luxembourg (1979) where figures are WHO estimates; Morocco (1971–1975) taken from the *United Nations demographic yearbook*.

females in Czechoslovakia also failed to show any improvement during the 1960s. But, again, since then death rates have fallen at all ages, leading to a gain of almost two years in life expectancy at birth over the past decade.

Mortality trends in Western and Southern Europe have tended to be much more uniform. Both sexes have enjoyed further gains in life expectancy at birth, although the improvement has been more impressive for females than for males. In addition, the most spectacular gains in longevity have occurred in countries of Southern Europe, with the result that the differential in life expectancy among countries of the European Region has narrowed considerably. Around 1960, for example, a male born in Sweden could expect to live roughly 10 years longer than his Portuguese counterpart; by 1980 this differential had been halved, with a similar relative change among females.

Given the variation in the reference periods used to construct life tables in the North African countries, plus the inconsistency of the sources used to compare the data, it is difficult to determine the true extent of improvements in mortality. However, it would appear that mortality among Algerian females, at least, has been declining during the 1970s even though only comparatively minor gains have been registered for males. In neighbouring Morocco, both males and females appear to have enjoyed gains of four to five years in life expectancy at birth during the 1960s. Indeed, a comparison based on experience around the early 1960s rather than on the decade 1962–1972 could well indicate even larger increments in life expectancy.

Age-specific mortality trends

Changes in life expectancy at birth reflect the net effect of trends in mortality at various ages. These changes may or may not be in the same direction. To gain insight into the complexity of the mortality changes that underlie these trends in life expectancy, the trends for selected countries chosen as being more or less representative of the patterns described above have been broken down into age components in Table 6. Very briefly, a lifetable methodology has been applied, which breaks down the changes in life expectancy at birth into the various age-specific contributions. A small overall interaction term is included which measures the total interactive effect of mortality change within each specific age group with that which occurs at higher ages.[a] It is obvious from Table 6 that the small net gain in life expectancy for males in the Netherlands since 1950 is largely attributable to further declines in infant and child mortality. Between the ages of 45 and 74, and especially at ages 55–74, male mortality has risen (as noted in the country report). This has tended to offset the gains in longevity resulting from improvements at the younger ages. Undoubtedly, much the same pattern of age contributions would emerge were the analysis to be repeated

---

[a] For a description of the methodology and a mathematical expression for the interaction term, *see* **Lopez, A.D. & Ruzicka, L.T.** The differential mortality of the sexes in Australia. *In*: McGlashan, N.D., ed. *Studies in Australian mortality.* Hobart, University of Tasmania, 1977 (Environmental Studies Occasional Paper No. 4), pp. 75–94.

Table 6. Age components of changing life expectancy at birth in selected countries, 1950–1954 to 1975–1978

Country	Life table periods	Sex	Contribution (in years) to change in life expectancy at birth due to mortality trends at ages:								Inter-action	Total increase in life expectancy (years)[a]
			0–14	15–24	25–34	35–44	45–54	55–64	65–74	75+		
England & Wales	1950–1954	M	1.37	0.06	0.21	0.20	0.25	0.42	0.24	0.19	0.09	3.0
	to	F	1.16	0.16	0.29	0.21	0.21	0.35	0.64	0.77	0.20	4.0
	1975–1978	F–M	-0.21	0.10	0.08	0.01	-0.04	-0.07	0.40	0.58	0.11	1.0
Hungary	1950–1954	M	2.83	0.33	0.29	0.30	0.41	0.27	0.18	0.18	0.16	4.9
	to	F	2.50	0.37	0.38	0.29	0.33	0.44	0.42	0.30	0.22	5.3
	1960–1964	F–M	-0.33	0.04	0.09	-0.01	-0.08	0.17	0.24	0.12	0.06	0.4
	1960–1964	M	1.49	0.08	-0.02	-0.30	-0.54	-0.27	-0.31	-0.12	0.01	0.0
	to	F	1.33	0.07	0.07	0.00	-0.06	-0.01	0.17	0.18	0.02	1.8
	1975–1978	F–M	-0.16	-0.01	0.09	0.30	0.48	0.26	0.48	0.30	0.01	1.8
Netherlands	1950–1954	M	1.51	0.00	0.15	0.10	-0.05	-0.33	-0.47	0.12	-0.01	1.0
	to	F	1.23	0.08	0.16	0.20	0.27	0.55	1.00	1.23	0.38	5.1
	1975–1978	F–M	-0.28	0.08	0.01	0.10	0.32	0.88	1.47	1.11	0.39	4.1

[a] The age components and the interaction contribution may not sum exactly to the total owing to rounding up.

Source: Computed from the WHO data bank.

for males in the Scandinavian countries. Females, too, have benefited from substantial declines in infant and child mortality and have continued to enjoy further reductions in death rates during middle age. It is also of interest to note the considerable improvement in mortality among elderly women in the Netherlands — roughly half of the total increase in life expectancy arose through mortality reductions at ages 65 and over.

Declines in infant and child mortality have also been responsible for much of the gain in life expectancy in England & Wales since the 1950s. Once again, in the case of females, this has been aided by a significant contribution from reductions in mortality among the elderly. In Hungary, on the other hand, a twofold analysis is shown, reflecting the marked alterations in mortality trends during the 1960s. Prior to that date, gains in life expectancy for both sexes were the result of lower mortality rates throughout life, but especially from those during infancy and childhood. Since 1960–1964, however, death rates for males at all ages beyond 25 years have increased, thus reducing life expectancy at birth. As Table 6 indicates, this trend has been exactly counterbalanced by further substantial declines in infant and child mortality, as well as by a slight improvement in mortality at ages 15–24 years. Interestingly, the analysis suggests that there has been no improvement and, in fact, a slight deterioration in adult female mortality over the last 15–20 years in Hungary. The gain in life expectancy that has been achieved for females has occurred almost entirely because of further declines in mortality at younger ages. A much smaller contribution has been made by lower death rates among the elderly.

Sex differentials in mortality

One of the most significant developments in mortality in the Region over the last quarter century or so is the widening gap in mortality between the sexes. The extent of concern with this problem is reflected by repeated reference to it in the country reports. Some idea of the age pattern of contributions to increasing excess male mortality can also be seen in Table 6. Thus, the 4.1-year increment in the sex mortality differential in the Netherlands since the early 1950s has arisen largely because of diverging mortality rates for men and women at ages 45 and over. The contribution from mortality changes at ages 0–14 has, however, acted to reduce the female advantage in life expectancy at birth over males. This reflects the greater absolute decline in mortality for males from the infective and parasitic diseases which were once common at these ages.[a] A somewhat similar pattern can be seen for Hungary where much of the recent increase in the sex mortality differential has arisen from a more widespread increase in mortality among adult males. Conversely, the comparatively small increment in male excess mortality in England & Wales since 1950 is almost entirely a reflection of greater reductions in mortality among elderly females. Mortality declines at other

[a] That male life expectancy has benefited more than that of females from the conquest of communicable diseases is due to the fact that the male death rate was higher at the time when the decline commenced.

ages, excluding young adulthood, have been of greater benefit to males. This would suggest that as the older cohorts die, the female advantage in life expectancy at birth in England & Wales may stabilize, or even begin to decrease should males continue to enjoy marginally higher gains in life expectancy during middle age.

A detailed analysis of the widening sex mortality differentials in neighbouring countries of the Region since the Second World War would almost certainly lead to similar conclusions, i.e. that the widespread failure of adult males to register further substantial declines in mortality is the dominant factor. When assessing the impact of the various causes of death on this trend, attention can therefore be restricted to those causes likely to be of greatest consequence at adult ages.[a]

The contribution of the leading causes of death to widening sex differentials among adults aged 35–74 can be seen in Table 7. For the developed countries as a whole, male excess mortality in this age group over the period since 1955–1959 has increased by about 157 deaths per 100 000 population. This is primarily because of differential mortality trends from heart disease and from cancer of the lung. In fact, these two causes alone accounted for over 80% of the change (based on this difference measure). Women also enjoyed a substantial advantage over men as the result of changing mortality from cerebrovascular diseases, cancer of the genital organs, and cirrhosis of the liver. For both sexes, death rates from cerebrovascular diseases have generally declined since the 1950s, and in some countries — such as the Netherlands and Sweden — a crossover in relative mortality has occurred with higher female death rates at the beginning of the period giving way gradually to excess male mortality. A similar effect can be seen for cancer of the genital organs, with women typically enjoying a marked reduction in mortality while the rate for males has remained unchanged, or even increased slightly in some countries.

Among the remaining causes shown in Table 7, only mortality from breast cancer and from violence (particularly from suicides and accidents other than those involving a motor vehicle) show a more favourable trend among males than females. Female death rates from breast cancer have generally increased since the Second World War, more so in Denmark, Hungary, Ireland and Italy. Much of the male advantage from trends in accident mortality, on the other hand, can be attributed to higher standards of industrial safety which, given the traditional sex division of labour, would have worked largely to the benefit of men. Suicide rates have also fallen recently for men in some countries (notably France and Sweden), but not for women. Indeed, female suicide rates in Hungary, Switzerland and some of the Northern European countries appear to have increased in recent years.

It is also of interest to review the contributory cause of death patterns for those nations showing the largest absolute increments in male excess

[a] Significant sex mortality differentials exist at other ages as well. In particular, male mortality at ages 15–24 in the developed countries of the Region is generally 2½–3 times the rate for females, due mostly to higher male mortality from traffic accidents.

Table 7. Contribution of various causes of death to the changing sex differential in mortality, 1955–1959 to 1975–1978

Cause of death	Titles in the A list of the ICD		Average contribution of cause to ΔSMD[a]		Countries with the largest absolute change per 100 000				
	Sixth and Seventh Revisions	Eighth Revision	per 100 000	%	Nether-lands	Hungary	Czecho-slovakia	Denmark	Sweden
All causes			157.3	100.0	370.3	352.8	290.2	274.4	273.1
Malignant neoplasms	A44–A59	A45–A60	59.0	37.5	132.4	95.3	97.1	47.9	49.5
of lung	A50	A51	39.4	25.0	92.4	57.6	62.8	39.2	21.7
of breast	A51	A54	-7.7	-4.9	-4.5	-17.4	-9.4	-5.8	0.6
of genital organs	A52–A54	A55–A57	12.7	8.1	11.0	25.6	14.1	14.0	12.1
Cardiovascular diseases	A79–A86	A80–A88	124.0	78.8	208.5	265.5	152.1	170.3	197.3
heart diseases	A79–A83	A80–A84	88.1	56.0	112.0	170.3	96.2	128.5	151.0
cerebrovascular diseases	A70	A85	26.5	16.8	30.3	67.5	47.0	27.3	34.8
Respiratory diseases	A87–A97	A89–A96	7.0	4.5	25.9	-6.2	54.1	34.5	15.9
Cirrhosis of the liver	A105	A102	12.9	8.2	4.3	19.2	28.0	18.1	16.2
Diabetes mellitus	A63	A64	5.8	3.7	10.1	-1.2	4.3	4.6	8.1
Violence	AE138–AE150	AE138–AE150	-4.1	-2.6	-11.2	48.6	15.8	-16.0	-4.6
motor vehicle accidents	AE138	AE138	0.4	0.3	-8.2	15.7	11.0	-8.8	-6.3
all other accidents	AE139–AE147	AE139–AE146	-4.5	-2.9	-5.1	13.8	-0.1	2.1	4.1
suicide	AE148	AE147	-2.9	-1.8	1.4	24.8	4.2	-9.5	-11.1
Senility and ill-defined	A136, A137	A136, A137	0.6	0.4	11.0	0.1	0.8	20.4	-1.2

[a] ΔSMD: change in the sex mortality differential over the period. Measured as the change in the male–female difference in age-standardized death rates for the age group 35–74 years. Excludes the experience of Bulgaria, the German Democratic Republic, Greece, Romania, Spain, the USSR and Yugoslavia, for which cause of death data were not available for the earlier period.

Source: Computed from the WHO data bank.

mortality. These are shown in the right hand columns of Table 7. Clearly, the diverging mortality of the sexes from cardiovascular diseases has been the primary determinant of recent changes in the sex differential. Among those countries of Northern and Eastern Europe for which the overall gap between the sexes has widened dramatically, roughly two thirds of the change — or about 200 excess male deaths per 100 000 population — can on average be attributed to these causes, especially to diseases of the heart.

The increment in the sex differential from other leading causes of death, particularly lung cancer and cerebrovascular disease, is also well above average in Czechoslovakia, Hungary and the Netherlands. Neither of these causes, however, has been particularly prominent in the trend towards higher male mortality in Denmark and Sweden. Rather, the impact of differential mortality trends from heart diseases would appear in itself to account for most of the change. Excess male mortality from violence, particularly from suicide, has declined in Denmark and Sweden since the 1950s, whereas in Czechoslovakia and Hungary the contribution from external causes has shown a tendency to increase in recent years.

Unfortunately, the heterogeneity of individual national structures precludes a more precise estimate of the significance of a single cause of death, or group of causes, for the changing sex pattern of mortality. Some trend characteristics for the various countries are worthy of note, however. In the Netherlands, for example, increasing excess male mortality from lung cancer is particularly evident, as is the contribution from respiratory diseases in Czechoslovakia. The widening gap in death rates between the sexes in Hungary since the 1950s can also be seen to be the result of a widespread increase in excess male mortality from most of the leading causes of death.

Infant and perinatal mortality

Given the substantial contribution of further declines in mortality at younger ages to the improvement in life expectancy in the European Region, it is perhaps appropriate at this point to consider these trends in somewhat greater detail. As one might expect, much of this contribution is the result of further reductions in infant mortality. The extent of these declines in selected countries of the Region can be seen in Table 8. A reduction of 50% or more in the infant mortality rate is apparent for most countries. The rate is currently at or below 8 deaths per 1000 live births in the Netherlands and in Scandinavia. This contrasts sharply with the experience of Algeria and Morocco, where an infant mortality rate of 130 per 1000 has not been uncommon. Some improvements in the urban areas of Morocco can be seen, however. The chances of infant survival have also improved markedly in Portugal, where the current rate of 26 deaths per 1000 live births is more in accord with regional experience. Much the same trend, though rather less exaggerated, can be discerned for perinatal mortality. This rate, in so far that stillbirths and early neonatal deaths are included in the denominator, is less subject to errors of definition and thus provides a more accurate appraisal of trends in endogenous causes of infant death.

Much of the decline in infant mortality has resulted from further reductions during the post-neonatal period when the infant, having survived

Table 8. Trends in infant and perinatal mortality in selected countries of the European Region, 1960–1980

Country	Perinatal mortality per 1000 live births			Infant mortality per 1000 live births		
	1960	1970	Around 1980	1960	1970	Around 1980
Algeria (North)				130.4	137.7	
Belgium[a]	28.4	20.4	15.9	26.7	17.9	13.1
Czechoslovakia	20.9	20.7	16.3	23.5	22.1	17.7
Finland	27.5		9.4	23.6		7.7
German Democratic Republic				38.8	18.5	12.1
Great Britain[a]				18.0[b]	15.0[c]	12.0
Greece	26.7	27.7	21.3	40.1	29.6	19.2
Hungary	35.5	34.5	23.1	47.6	35.9	23.2
Luxembourg[a]				23.4	22.0	11.1
Morocco		71.0		134.6[d]	96.0[d]	
Netherlands[a]	24.1[e]	17.2[e]	10.2[e]	15.7	11.1	7.4
Norway	22.5[b]	16.4[c]	11.1[f]	17.1[b]	11.6[c]	8.1[f]
Portugal	41.1	37.0	31.3[g]	77.5	55.5	26.0[f]
Sweden	26.2	16.4	8.7	16.6	11.0	6.9

[a] Rates are for females only.

[b] 1961–1965.

[c] 1971–1975.

[d] Urban areas only.

[e] Perinatal mortality ratio (includes late fetal deaths in the denominator).

[f] Provisional.

[g] 1975.

Source: Respective country reports except for Luxembourg, where figures for 1960 and 1970 have been taken from the *United Nations demographic yearbook*. The 1978 figure for Luxembourg is the author's estimate calculated from data given in the *United Nations demographic yearbook*.

the constitutional "test" so to speak, is exposed to environmental hazards. In Great Britain, for example, post-neonatal mortality is now about one third of its level immediately following the Second World War. Neonatal deaths (those occurring in the first month of life) fell by about 50% during the same period. According to the country report, "the decline in the post-neonatal death rate has been caused by the reduction in deaths from infective and parasitic diseases, enteritis and other diarrhoeal diseases and in deaths from respiratory disease. These deaths which are associated with environmental factors have become much less important in comparison with deaths due to congenital malformations and birth injuries which amounted to over two thirds of all infant deaths in 1975". Undoubtedly, much the same structural change underlies the trends in other countries as well.

Given that the health of the newborn is particularly sensitive to environmental conditions, the infant mortality rate (more accurately, the post-neonatal mortality rate) is widely regarded as a good indicator of the social and economic environment of the infant, and is taken to reflect the availability and efficacy of infant health care as well. Variations in infant mortality rates among and within countries may then be interpreted as indicators of differences in the underlying health environment of infants. According to the Finnish report, illegitimate children have significantly higher infant and perinatal mortality rates than legitimate infants, identifying them as a particular risk group. Babies with low birth weight, the cause of which may be predominantly socioeconomic, also experience higher mortality than those weighing 2500 grammes or more at birth. In Hungary, for example, data for 1980 suggest that the infant mortality rate for the latter group is 8.2 per 1000 compared with a rate of 153 per 1000 for babies whose weight at birth was below this threshold. Moreover, about 11% of births in Hungary are premature, and little change has occurred in this proportion over the last decade at least.

As one might expect, the largest differentials in infant mortality are to be found in the North African countries, where the level of socioeconomic development is less advanced and overall mortality is correspondingly higher. In rural areas, unsanitary traditional birth practices still prevail in many societies, and adequate health care facilities are generally lacking. As a consequence, infant and child mortality in these areas is usually well in excess of that found in the cities. This pattern is confirmed from the findings for Algeria and Morocco. According to the latest available data (referring to the latter part of the 1960s) infant mortality in rural areas of Algeria was around 133 per 1000 live births, compared with a rate of about 113 per 1000 in the cities. In Morocco, the corresponding rates were 170 and 120 per 1000 respectively.

Socioeconomic and regional mortality differentials

In Chapter 4 reference is made to the marked socioeconomic differentials in mortality that exist in the developed countries, with those in the lowest social strata suffering the greatest risks to health. These findings need not be repeated here, though mention should be made of some of the more significant social, economic and regional differentials in mortality reported in the individual country studies. In Finland, for example, where the urban/rural differential in mortality is slight, significant geographical differences still exist. Life expectancy in the eastern and northern parts of the country is somewhat lower than in southern and western Finland. The Finnish report goes on to note that this division is roughly consistent with the linguistic pattern of the country, with male mortality being considerably lower in the Swedish-speaking municipalities. This suggests that there may be a predominant behavioural explanation for geographical differences since male mortality in Sweden, in sharp contrast to that in Finland, is one of the lowest in the world. In the Netherlands, by far the highest death rates for both males and females (7–16% above the national average) are to be found in the provinces of Limburg — a major mining area until quite recently — and North Brabant, suggesting a clear environmental impact on health. A similar finding is reported for Norway, where the old manufacturing countries were found to have a higher than average mortality. Moreover, in Norway there is evidence of regional differentials in mortality that are independent of the degree of urbanization; the northern part of Norway experiences markedly higher death rates than the southern counties, with the exception of Oslo.

According to a recent study of mortality in Greece, death rates from almost all causes were higher in the urban centres. Only certain sites of cancer (stomach and skin), nutritional deficiencies, infectious diseases and suicide show higher death rates in rural districts. As the Greek report concludes, "these findings suggest that the better medical care (and presumably the lower fatality rates) in the urban population is unable to overcome the higher incidence of many serious diseases in this population, and indicate a need for a change of emphasis in program planning in preventive medicine".

Studies on occupational mortality in Norway show relatively low mortality for teachers and farmers, and comparatively high death rates for seamen and for restaurant and hotel employees. It is interesting to note that the Norwegian report ascribes these differences largely to lifestyle factors. However, the contribution from occupational risks, especially in relation to accidents among seamen, is also recognized. Substantial occupational differences in mortality were also reported for Algeria, where children born to families where neither parent had a profession could expect to live, on average, for some 13 years less than their counterparts born into families where at least one parent was either an employee, a merchant, or a managerial worker. Similarly, the chances of infant survival in Algeria are affected by the educational level of the head of household. Thus, a child born to a family where the head of household is literate can expect to live about 10 years longer than one born into an illiterate household, with the disparity between the two groups being greatest in urban areas.

With advances in medical technology, infectious and parasitic diseases have been greatly reduced in the European Region. The southern extremity is an exception. The focus of public health concern has increasingly shifted towards chronic diseases such as coronary heart disease and lung cancer, which account for the overwhelming majority of deaths in the Region and to which adult males in particular appear to be especially susceptible. Epidemiological research has consistently identified detrimental lifestyle practices — prominent among which is cigarette smoking — in the etiology of these diseases. This suggests that greater emphasis should be placed on behaviour modification programmes within health strategies designed to cope with them.

Intra-European migration

Population composition, and indeed the very forces of natural demographic change, can be significantly influenced by the geographical movement of individuals. Over the last quarter of a century or so, new and complex patterns of intra-European migration have emerged. These, in terms of the magnitude of the flows, have often had a significant impact on the labour force structure of both the host country and the country of origin. Furthermore, although the majority of migrants probably leave their native country with the intention of returning to it, many eventually remain abroad and currently they constitute sizeable minorities in the major host countries. Moreover, migrants generally predominate among the poorer echelons of society, in part because of cultural differences. As a result, migrants are confronted with special problems related to living and working conditions, education and health. It is imperative, therefore, that the host country recognizes and acts to alleviate these problems, thus reducing social tensions and facilitating the process of assimilation.

Overview of regional migration streams

With the rapid economic growth in Western Europe during the late 1950s, the demand for labour in many countries could no longer be satisfied locally. Consequently it became necessary to recruit foreign workers. The main sources of supply were the countries bordering the Mediterranean basin where economic development was less advanced and where rapid population growth had been the norm. The geographical pattern of contemporary European migration can, therefore, be attributed largely to differential demographic and economic growth.

The magnitude of these population movements can be gauged from various estimates of the numbers of foreign workers in the receiving countries at different times. For instance the International Labour Office (ILO)[a] has estimated that in the early 1970s the European Community countries, Austria, Norway, Sweden and Switzerland together employed some 7.5 million foreign workers. According to the United Nations,[b] about 5.5 million immigrants from Southern Europe were living in countries of the northern

[a] *Some growing employment problems in Europe.* Geneva, International Labour Office, 1973.

[b] *Trends and characteristics of international migration since 1950.* New York, United Nations, 1979 (Demographic Studies No. 64).

and western regions of the continent in 1974. Since that data, however, intra-European labour migration has fallen sharply, primarily as a result of economic recession but also because of increasing concern in the host countries about their ability to absorb what are already considerable foreign minorities. The main immigration countries — Belgium, France, the Federal Republic of Germany, the Netherlands, Sweden and Switzerland — have all subsequently imposed more strict controls on the intake of migrants. In fact, data from some emigration countries — including Algeria, Greece and Italy — indicate a reversal of migration trends in specific years because of the return of migrant workers.

Table 9 summarizes the migration experience of the different regions of Europe from 1950. The contrast between the strong positive balance of migration in Western Europe and the substantial losses experienced by countries in the southern part of the region is particularly striking. One should also note the marked decline in net emigration from Eastern Europe. Although the migration of workers is by no means a new phenomenon in Europe, the exchange between countries with surplus labour and those with a labour demand reached unprecedented levels in the last few decades. The actual gross movements, however, are difficult to measure since the statistics of most countries tend to understate the number of departing workers. Despite this bias, evidence from several European countries indicates that the gross annual movement of foreign labour is typically about four times the net figure. This would suggest that contemporary labour migration within Europe is to a large extent temporary, many workers returning home after a few years to be replaced by others and/or re-emigrating at a later date.

National migration flows

From an inspection of the migration data for the individual countries of Western Europe, it is clear that France and the Federal Republic of Germany contribute most to the large positive balance. During each of the three periods under review, France and the Federal Republic alone accounted for 98%, 86% and 87%, respectively, of the overall net gain for the region. This is not to imply, however, that these two countries also had the highest net migration rates. This distinction belonged to Switzerland until 1960, and to Luxembourg from 1960 onwards. The impact of migration has been particularly noticeable in the latter country, where currently no less than 26% of the entire population is foreign-born. In Switzerland, too, the supply of indigenous labour has lagged far behind demand. According to ILO estimates, migrant workers comprised some 30% of the Swiss labour force by the end of 1973. This is about 2½–3 times more than in France and the Federal Republic of Germany.

Because of the large number of refugees (about 8 million) from the East, the Federal Republic of Germany had little need to import labour until the end of the 1950s. Immediately thereafter labour shortages became acute, and a remarkable number of "guest workers" were recruited in the space of a couple of years. Some 700 000 foreign nationals were recorded in the 1961 census, and almost 200 000 of them came from Italy. The formation of the

Table 9. Net migration in Europe, 1960–1974[a]

Region of Europe[b]	Estimated net migration			Average annual net migration per 1000 population		
	1950–1960	1960–1970	1970–1974	1950–1960	1960–1970	1970–1974
Northern	-500 000	-278 000	-83 000	-0.7	-0.4	-0.3
Western	3 705 000	4 919 000	2 235 000	2.9	3.5	3.7
Eastern	-2 741 000	-1 031 000	-158 000	-3.0	-1.0	-0.4
Southern	-3 475 000	-3 676 000	-1 083 000	-3.1	-3.1	-2.1

[a] Estimates based on mid-year population.

[b] As defined by the United Nations. See note to Table 1.

Source: *Trends and characteristics of international migration since 1950.* New York, United Nations, 1979 (Demographic Studies No. 64).

European Economic Community (EEC), with a treaty ensuring the right of free movement of labour, greatly facilitated Italian emigration. Of the initial six EEC members, Italy was the only one with a labour surplus. However, as Italy itself was undergoing rapid industrialization it clearly could not satisfy the labour needs of the rest of the Community for long. The appearance of new sources of labour is reflected in the 1970 census in the Federal Republic. By that year the foreign population had increased to 2.6 million, the predominant nationalities being Turkish and Yugoslav followed by Greek, Italian and Spanish. As a consequence of economic recession, the recruitment of workers from outside the EEC (except for a small number of occupations) ceased in the Federal Republic in 1973. The majority of immigrants subsequently admitted have been family members of foreigners already settled there.

In France, despite nearly a million French nationals returning from Algeria in the early 1960s, the annual intake of foreign workers grew more or less continuously during the 1950s and 1960s, reaching 255 000 in 1970. As with other European Community members, France initially relied heavily on Italy to meet its growing labour needs. By the beginning of the 1960s, however, Spain had replaced Italy as the main source of foreign workers in France, and since the mid-1960s, Portugal has taken over this role. The fear of economic recession, however, subsequently led to the suspension of migration (with certain exceptions) in July 1974.

Belgium, like France, has for many decades encouraged the permanent settlement of foreign migrants to compensate for a low rate of natural population growth. The net migration gain for this comparatively small country amounted to about 240 000 people between 1960 and 1969. Despite stricter immigration controls since the mid-1970s, the net gain for the period 1970–1977 was still considerable (176 000). At the time of the 1961 census there were already more than 200 000 Italians living in Belgium, and as late as 1977 they were still by far the most dominant group. New trends in migration did, however, develop during this period. For example, the yearly intake of Moroccans and Turks expanded from a few hundred in 1961 to 81 000 and 59 000, respectively, in 1977. Currently, about one tenth of the total Belgian population are aliens, about half of whom reside in the French-speaking region of the country. The remainder are roughly equally dispersed between the Flemish areas outside Brussels and the capital itself. Furthermore, the distribution within Brussels reveals a strong concentration of foreigners in the inner city; some 60% of all immigrants living in the capital are found in 5 of the 19 communes constituting the Brussels agglomeration.

In contrast to its neighbours, the Netherlands has witnessed substantial population movements only since the 1960s. During that decade the net annual gain from the migration of non-Dutch nationals was around 14 000. At the same time, however, the external migration balance of Dutch nationals continued to be negative, so that the total migration surplus in fact halved. Most immigrants who entered the Netherlands during the 1960s were from the Mediterranean countries, and were usually single or unaccompanied males. As a consequence of diminishing demand, the migration policy was changed in 1974, and immigration during the second half of the 1970s has been dominated by family reunification. This is reflected in the occupational composition of immigrants: the proportion of immigrants without an occupation at the time of entry increased from 47% in 1970 to 73% in 1979.

Population pressures and economic considerations have long encouraged emigration in most Mediterranean countries. Current labour migrations may, therefore, be viewed as the continuation of a long established trend, with only the destination countries changing over recent decades. According to 1979 United Nations estimates, net losses from emigration during the 1950–1974 period totalled 2.2 million in Portugal, 2.0 million in Italy, 1.7 million in Spain, 1.6 million in Yugoslavia and 650 000 in Greece. Switzerland has been the leading destination for Italian migration within Europe, attracting some 40% of all Italians emigrating between 1950 and 1974. France, on the other hand, has been the choice of four out of every five Portuguese emigrants moving to another country in Europe. Figures for Portugal indicate that the number of persons leaving the country increased from 33 000 in 1960 to 173 000 in 1970. Since then emigration, and particularly clandestine emigration, has fallen rapidly so that by 1980 the total number of departures was barely 21 000.

The overwhelming majority of Greek continental migrants have moved to the Federal Republic of Germany which, during the 1960s, was the destination of more than half a million Greeks. As a consequence of growing employment opportunities at home and restrictions on immigration imposed by the major receiving countries, the number of emigrants fell sharply after 1970. The latest available migration figures, which include intercontinental emigration, indicate that a little over 16 500 people left the country in 1977 while roughly 12 500 entered it. Interestingly, the proportion of male migrants in each of the two flows has decreased since 1960 which, as noted in the country report, no doubt signifies the characteristic time-lag between the migration of married men and that of their families.

Conditions within the Maghreb countries have long encouraged emigration. The present geographical pattern of movement, with France as the main destination, obviously reflects colonial links. This is especially evident in the case of Algeria; 90% of all overseas residents are thought to be living in France. As mentioned earlier, the annual rates of population growth are extremely high in Morocco and Algeria, with the result that many young workers who enter the labour market each year are unable to find employment. Traditionally, males have constituted the vast majority of migrants, with an increasing proportion under 25 years of age. Since the end of the 1960s, however, the tendency has been for those who are married to send for their families. The increasing trend towards family migration is evident from the returns of the 1975 French census. This revealed that one third of the Algerians living in France were women. The number of Algerians living overseas has continued to rise since independence in 1962. At that time, some 335 000 were already living in France. By the time immigration was suspended in 1973, more than 800 000 Algerians had taken up residence in France. Since then, migration statistics indicate that more Algerians have returned home than have emigrated. This has not, however, reduced the size of the Algerian population in France; in 1978 this was estimated still to be around one million.

The net migration figures presented in Table 9 for Northern Europe conceal the considerable heterogeneity of national migration patterns, especially between the Scandinavian countries and Ireland and the United Kingdom. As Table 10 illustrates, the migration experience of these two areas is quite distinct. While it is well known that Ireland has been a country of emigration for many years, the United Kingdom is more often than not perceived as a nation that has received large waves of immigrants. In reality, the situation in the United Kingdom is more complex, since concurrent with this inward movement it has also traditionally supplied migrant stock to North America, Australia and New Zealand in particular. According to the British report, about 2.6 million people emigrated from Great Britain and 2.1 million settlers were admitted from abroad during the period 1967–1976. Prior to 1962, labour shortages and economic expansion attracted many migrants from the newly independent countries of the Commonwealth.

The predominance of Commonwealth citizens among migrants to the United Kingdom continued throughout the period 1966–1976. During this

Table 10. Net migration estimates for Northern Europe by major regions, 1950–1974

Region	1950–1960	1960–1970	1970–1974
Scandinavia	-46 000	64 000	54 000
Ireland and the United Kingdom	-454 000	-342 000	-137 000

Source: *Trends and characteristics of international migration since 1950.* New York, United Nations, 1979 (Demographic Studies No. 64).

time they accounted for close to 60% of all non-Irish immigrants. A more detailed examination of the annual pattern of British migration reveals that immigrants from the New Commonwealth countries constitute the major share (60%) of those of Commonwealth origin. Conversely, three quarters of the emigrants who left Britain between 1966 and 1976 for a Commonwealth destination went to the Old Commonwealth, particularly to Australia. On the whole, some 60% of the total emigration flow during this period was to other Commonwealth countries. However, as a result of increasing unemployment, the Australian and New Zealand governments have recently reduced their migrant intake. Consequently in 1975, for the first time ever, more British emigrants went to non-Commonwealth countries than to those in the Commonwealth. Whether this is merely a temporary change rather than an emerging pattern of migration remains to be seen.

Among the Nordic countries, Sweden alone has seen large-scale immigration. With the exception of 1972 and 1973, Sweden has consistently had a positive migration balance with other countries since the end of the Second World War. Between 1950 and 1970 the trend in immigration was clearly upward, and the net intake for the period 1965–1969 totalled about 128 000. The deceleration of economic growth in Sweden, as elsewhere, during the early 1970s resulted in a sharp decline in immigration: the net gain over the period 1970–1974 fell to around 38 000 persons. During the last five years, however, immigration has once again been allowed to increase, resulting in a surplus of 80 000 people. Moreover, in view of the 1954 agreement permitting the free movement of labour among the Nordic countries, it is perhaps not surprising that Danes, Finns and Norwegians predominate among immigrants to Sweden. Indeed, during the 1950s and 1960s, Finns alone accounted for over 50% of Swedish net migration. Of the remainder, Greeks and Yugoslavs have become increasingly dominant in the migration flow to Sweden, especially since the mid-1960s.

Towards the end of the 1960s, the Swedish government introduced stricter controls on non-Nordic immigration. As a result, the share of migrants from other European countries fell from 31% in 1972 to 22% in 1980. At the same time, the intake of refugees grew sharply, resulting in a threefold increase in the number of Asian and South American immigrants during the 1970s.

In contrast to the other Nordic countries, Finland has been a major supplier of migrants. According to 1979 United Nations estimates, more than half a million Finns had left the country since the end of the Second World War. Although many subsequently returned, the net loss (270 000) during that period nonetheless amounted to 5.5% of the total population of the country. The main recipients of Finnish emigrants over the last 20 years have been Australia, Canada, New Zealand, Sweden and the United States. Peak emigration occurred towards the end of the 1960s, reaching 40 000 in each of two consecutive years (1969 and 1970). Since then, the annual number of emigrants has varied between 10 000 and 20 000. At the same time, however, the number of immigrants has remained relatively high, leading to a positive balance for the period 1971–1975. Interestingly, the vast majority of immigrants to Finland are nationals returning from Sweden; in 1979, for instance, this group accounted for more than 85% of new settlers.

Prior to the mid-1960s the Norwegian migration balance remained negative, and it was not until 1970 that Norway experienced net immigration of any significance. Since then, the average number of persons entering the country with the intention of settling has been around 19 000, resulting in a net average gain of about 4000 per year. The countries with which Norway has generally had the greatest migration exchange include Denmark, Sweden, the United Kingdom and the United States. Since 1971, however, many Pakistanis and citizens of other Asian countries have been permitted to enter Norway, and they currently account for about one third of the annual net intake.

According to the migration figures given in the Czechoslovakian report, the average annual number of emigrants since 1960 has varied between 3000 and 4000. An exception was 1970, with more than 12 000 persons emigrating, all but 760 of whom were from the Czech Socialist Republic. This composition in fact is not inconsistent with previous experience indicating that emigration rates for the Slovak Socialist Republic are generally well below those of the Czech Socialist Republic. Furthermore, the number of people emigrating is usually far in excess of those immigrating, although 1973 was an exception; in that year a net migration gain of 1777 was recorded.

In general, however, given the absence of information about countries of origin and destination in migration statistics, comparatively little is known about the nature and patterns of external migration in Eastern Europe. Drawing on various sources, it would appear that bilateral agreements have resulted in a considerable short-term exchange of workers between the socialist countries. The German Democratic Republic seems to be the main labour importing country, employing some 13 000 Hungarian, 12 000 Polish and 2000 Czechoslovakian workers in recent years.[a] Indeed, according to

---

[a] *Trends and characteristics of international migration since 1950.* New York, United Nations, 1979 (Demographic Studies No. 64). *See also* **Compton, P.** Migration in Eastern Europe. *In*: Salt, J. & Clout, H., ed. *Migration in post-war Europe.* London, Oxford University Press, 1976.

ILO, these imbalances in the labour market are likely to increase in the future and may well necessitate even greater external migration among the Eastern European countries.

Internal migration

In many respects, the distinction between external and internal migration is an artificial one since the two forms of mobility are closely related. In a recent report[a] the United Nations Economic Commission for Europe stressed the close links that exist "between internal migration, the changing needs for labour and international migration". Indeed, much of the international labour migration referred to in the previous section would not have occurred had available reserves of labour still existed in the rural areas of the recipient countries. A particularly pervasive trend has been the clustering of population into a few principal centres in each country. Rapid urbanization is largely a consequence of the process of industrialization which, in turn, has depended on labour drawn from the countryside, often leading to the depopulation of rural and remote areas. An attendant cost of this process has been the exacerbation of regional disparities in income, opportunities and living standards, all of which have further encouraged people to move. As overall population growth has slackened in most European countries, the issue of internal migration has received greater prominence and it increasingly forms an integral part of regional policy. Migration is a highly selective process which, in addition to its short-term impact on population size, also affects the age structure and, more often than not, the sex composition of the local population. In the longer term, therefore, migration may also be expected to exert an effect on the process of natural change arising from births and deaths.

An internal migration is generally defined as a move made from one area to another during a given period and involving a permanent change of residence within a country. For the purposes of this study, a distinction is also made between highly localized moves, often referred to as residential mobility, and moves over longer distances whereby migrants simultaneously change their place of residence and their employment. The latter type usually involves crossing a local or regional boundary, and has a different social and economic dimension. This form of migration, in fact, forms part of the process of socioeconomic change and is usually closely related to underlying societal transformations.

Western Europe, one of the most urbanized regions in the world, has long witnessed substantial flows of migrants from the countryside to the cities. This movement still predominates in the less developed parts of Europe. In the more highly industrialized and urbanized parts, however, other factors have emerged that in many cases have reversed the traditional balance of migration. Thus, during the period following the Second World War a continuation of the movement from declining rural regions to growing

[a] *Labour supply and migration in Europe: demographic dimensions 1950–1975 and prospects.* Geneva, United Nations, 1979.

industrial and commercial centres can be seen in some regions, being especially common in Eastern and Southern Europe. A second type of spatial mobility, which accounts for an ever increasing share of total migrations, is the movement between urban zones and, more recently, a flow out from the centre of major towns. These types of move are mostly characteristic of Western and Northern Europe. A third emerging pattern that can be distinguished is the interregional flow resulting from variable employment opportunities and/or environmental attractions, and is especially apparent in Western Europe.

Urbanization

Some idea of the extent of population redistribution and urbanization in Europe can be gained from Table 11. In 1950 more than half of the total population lived in urban areas; 25 years later this proportion had increased to 67%. The growth in the size of the urban population, in relative terms at least, has been greatest in Southern Europe where it more than doubled over the period. In Northern Europe, on the other hand, where the process of urbanization was already well advanced by the middle of the century, the increase has been comparatively small; the urban population has grown by about one quarter. Interestingly, along with Southern Europe, the largest relative declines in the size of the rural population have occurred in Western Europe. As a consequence of these trends, the interregional variation in the degree of urbanization has diminished. In 1950 the difference between the least (Southern Europe) and most (Northern Europe) urbanized regions amounted to 32 percentage points; by 1975 this gap had been reduced by about half.

Considerable caution, however, must be exercised when interpreting such changes. To begin with, it is exceedingly difficult to measure the real amount of rural–urban migration. Apart from the fact that there is no internationally recognized definition of "rural" and "urban", other factors such as compensatory flows must be taken into account. These may, for example, include elderly people returning to the countryside, or urban workers who prefer to live in rural surroundings and who commute to their work in a nearby city. This is of particular significance in a country like Luxembourg, where in 1970 close to 40% of the total workforce lived in a different commune (administrative unit) to the one in which they worked.

Despite these caveats, it is nevertheless clear that most rural communities in Europe have experienced heavy emigration since the end of the Second World War. This is also reflected in occupational statistics. These reveal that some 30 million people in the EEC in 1950 were engaged in primary activities, whereas by 1972 the figure had fallen to less than 8.5 million. Moreover, this trend is also characteristic of countries where a large proportion of the workforce has traditionally been involved in farming, fishing and forestry. In Portugal and Spain, where roughly half of the workforce in 1950 was engaged in these occupations, the proportions had fallen to 31% and 29%, respectively, by 1972.

The predominant type of migration in Southern Europe has been movement from rural to urban areas. In Greece, for example, 45% of all

Table 11. Urban–rural population change in Europe between 1950 and 1975

		Index of population change (1950 = 100)			Percentage of population living in urban areas
		Total	Urban	Rural	
Northern Europe	1950	100	100	100	68
	1975	114	126	89	75
Western Europe	1950	100	100	100	63
	1975	124	153	76	77
Eastern Europe[a]	1950	100	100	100	43
	1975	121	159	92	57
Southern Europe	1950	100	100	100	36
	1975	122	204	77	59
Total	1950	100	100	100	52
	1975	121	157	82	67

[a] Excluding the USSR.

Source: *Trends and characteristics of international migration since 1950.* New York, United Nations, 1979 (Demographic Studies No. 64).

migrations between 1965 and 1971 were of this type, and the net urban gain was around 264 000.[a] This pattern also dominates the flows in the Maghreb countries and often represents the first step towards international migration. This has, for example, been the case in Algeria where the large centres such as Algiers, Oran, Constantine and Sunaba have, since independence, experienced intense migration from the rural districts.

The extensive economic, social and political transformations that have taken place in Eastern Europe since the Second World War have been accompanied by a high level of geographical mobility. Although agriculture remains of much greater significance than in the economies of Western Europe, a substantial amount of labour has been released from the land and has moved to other types of employment in the cities. As a consequence, the urban population has expanded rapidly in these countries with the notable exceptions of Czechoslovakia and the German Democratic Republic, where as early as 1950 roughly half the population were living in urban areas. One must also recognize that the nature of the flows will be affected by the degree to which the country is urbanized (Table 12). Thus in Hungary, the least urbanized of the three countries, rural to rural migration still accounted for

[a] *Trends and characteristics of international migration since 1950.* New York, United Nations, 1979 (Demographic Studies No. 64).

Table 12. Urban/rural flows of internal migration

Country	Total internal migration (thousands)	Percentage of total flow moving from:				Total
		urban to urban	rural to urban	urban to rural	rural to rural	
Czechoslovakia						
1963–1964	800	38	30	13	19	100
1970–1971	799	37	31	14	18	100
German Democratic Republic						
1963–1964	1528	54	21	14	11	100
1970–1972	1198	49	24	14	13	100
Hungary						
1960–1964	1654	10	29	15	46	100
1970–1974	1293	11	30	16	43	100

Source: *Trends and characteristics of international migration since 1950.* New York, United Nations, 1979 (Demographic Studies No. 64).

more than 40% of total migration while inter-urban flows were comparatively small. This contrasts sharply with the internal migration distributions in Czechoslovakia and the German Democratic Republic, where some 70% of all migrants had an urban destination.

With regard to the intensity of migration in Eastern Europe, there has been a marked decline in mobility with the restructuring of the economies towards secondary and tertiary activities. Compton,[a] for instance, has estimated that some 2.1 million people migrated between settlements in Bulgaria, Czechoslovakia, the German Democratic Republic, Hungary and Poland in 1970, whereas 15 years earlier the number of migrants within these same countries was approximately twice as large. According to Hungarian data, for example, the absolute number of migrations fell by about 40% between 1960 and 1980. Part of this decline is attributable to a decrease in the volume of movement to Budapest which had dominated the pattern in the 1960s. On the other hand, the Czechoslovakian migration data suggest that spatial mobility levels stabilized in Czechoslovakia in the early 1970s. Since then, the annual rate of internal movement appears to have fluctuated between 25 and 30 migrants per 1000 population. As was found for international migration, those living in the Czech Socialist Republic were also more mobile within the country than their Slovak counterparts.

[a] **Compton, P.** Migration in Eastern Europe. *In*: Salt, J. & Clout, H., ed. *Migration in post-war Europe.* London, Oxford University Press, 1976.

Inter-urban flows and "the flight from the cities"

In Western and Northern Europe almost all long-distance migration is inter-urban and, although the volume of population exchange between these areas may be considerable, the net gain or loss is usually quite small. Richmond,[a] in discussing the complex nature of migration in post-industrial society, has made a number of interesting observations about such flows. In particular, he notes that the demographic and occupational characteristics of inter-urban migrants are almost identical. Thus, in spite of the large gross exchanges involved, the structural characteristics of the urban populations remain largely unaffected. Moreover, contemporary migration flows are only in part governed by distance. Of much greater significance is the lure of better opportunities perceived to be available at the place of destination. In Richmond's view, the traditional search for "push" or "pull" factors is no longer realistic since "migration, like other forms of occupational and social mobility, has become a functional imperative in advanced industrial societies".

According to the 1961 census of Great Britain, more than 60% of internal moves were between urban areas. Although the predominance of inter-city flows has not changed in later censuses, there has been a growing tendency for city dwellers to move to rural areas. The first stage of population decentralization, which has been particularly characteristic of the older and larger agglomerations, was the movement away from the city centre to new suburbs and satellite towns. Recently, this growth appears to have halted with a concomitant increase in the proportion of the population living in rural areas. This movement, however, should not be interpreted as a sign of rural renaissance but rather represents a blurring of the distinction between rural and urban lifestyles. Indeed, with the improvement in commuting facilities, many of those who work in a city nowadays prefer to live elsewhere.

In Belgium, the continuing depopulation of the cities, according to the country report, occurs largely from the departure of Belgians. Most of the areas vacated in Brussels, however, have subsequently been inhabited by foreign workers and their families. Similarly, the Dutch internal migration pattern during the period 1960–1979 shows a clear shift in the direction of net migration at the regional level. Population losses in the northern provinces and in Zealand have been reversed with these areas currently experiencing a net gain. Conversely, losses from migration are still apparent in the highly urbanized zones of northern and southern Holland.

In Scandinavia, too, a number of significant changes have occurred in the pattern of internal migration during the 1970s. Prior to 1970 in Sweden there had been a substantial movement of people to the urban agglomerations, primarily from the rural areas in the north and north-western parts of the country. Since then, there has been a reversal of this trend with

---

[a] **Richmond, A.H.** Sociology of migration in industrial and post-industrial societies. *In*: Jackson, J.A., ed. *Migration.* Cambridge, Cambridge University Press, 1969 (Sociological Studies No. 2).

Stockholm, for example, experiencing net migration losses throughout the 1970s. At the same time, there has been a slackening in the total internal migration level. A similar decline in overall mobility is apparent for Norway since 1975. Further, as a result of outflows from Oslo's central districts, the migration balance altered quite markedly during the 1966–1970 period. The population losses of Oslo are thought to have been largely a consequence of poor housing, although this is probably true for many other large agglomerations. The two most common types of internal migrant in Norway are single people in their early twenties, who move to the larger urban centres, and those in their thirties who move out of the major cities with their families.

The migration patterns in Finland over the period 1960–1980 indicate that there has been a consistent net inflow to the southern provinces; the eastern and northern parts of the country have, however, witnessed net outflow. The level of migration over this period varied between 40 and 58 migrants per 1000 population. There is evidence to suggest that the attraction of southern Finland, and of Helsinki in particular, has diminished in recent years. A comparison of the occupational structure of Finnish internal migrants with that of the total workforce indicates a relative excess of professional, technical, administrative, managerial and clerical workers among migrants. This is consistent with the findings of other migration studies and is usually attributed to the fact that workers in these occupations are often employed by large public or private multi-locational organizations. Many individuals, therefore, move as a result of career promotion or transfer. Another factor that contributes to their high spatial mobility is the specialized nature of many of these occupations. One consequence of this is that the demand for their skills extends beyond the immediate locality to the national and occasionally international level. Moving for this group is thus often a "functional necessity" and, in many cases, represents the only means of advancing their careers. The occupational categories that tend to be under-represented in the migration flows are, not surprisingly, those connected with the exploitation of natural resources such as farming, fishing, etc.

Finally, it is worthwhile mentioning that the British report contains a number of interesting predictions about future trends in internal migration, which may be applicable to other parts of Western and Northern Europe. In particular, the shift away from the larger metropolitan areas is expected to continue. On the other hand, increasing commuting costs may well mitigate the current rates of decentralization. Moreover, with the declining growth of national populations and further migration losses among the older inner-city districts, governments may be increasingly pressured into providing greater assistance for the regeneration of these areas. This course of action may be expected to stem the volume of outflow in the future; and it may even lead to a reversal of net migration from the city core in due course.

Some Health and Social Implications

The consequences of demographic change for the health and social services may essentially be viewed as arising in two interdependent ways. First, there is the recognition that demographic trends in the European Region — and in particular the trends in mortality — depend closely on social norms and behavioural traits and are often manifested through a dose–response relationship. For example, future mortality trends up to the year 2000 can already be predicted in the case of lung cancer with reasonable certainty from knowledge of previous smoking habits.[a] Second, the momentum of population growth is largely determined by the age structure of the population. This in turn reflects past trends in fertility, and to a lesser extent in mortality and migration. In some cases, appropriate and effective health education and intervention strategies can be expected to alter the course of demographic change. The recent decline in mortality from coronary heart disease, for example, would appear to be in large part the result of education-inspired behaviour modifications and the more efficacious treatment of coronary patients.

Future population composition

Perhaps the more widely recognized implications of demographic trends are those that are reflected through population composition, particularly with regard to age, sex and geographical distribution. Indeed, it is the health and social consequences of the future population age structure that draws most comment in the country reports. In this respect, the expected further increase in the number and proportion of the elderly is the most dominant feature. The number of people aged 60 and over in Hungary, for example, is expected to be 11% greater by the turn of the century. Similarly, the proportion aged 65 and over is expected to rise by more than a third in the Netherlands, with the excess of females increasing from 34.5% to 44.8% under the most likely conditions. In both Greece and Luxembourg this same age group will account for about 14% of the total population in the year 2000, some three percentage points more than was the case in the early 1970s.

More specific age projections of the elderly population reveal, however, that the actual situation is likely to be somewhat more complex. In Great Britain, the number of people of pensionable age is expected to continue to increase, but at a slower rate, until 1991. During the 1990s, though, the smaller birth cohorts of the 1920s and 1930s will reach pensionable age and as a result this population is projected to decline to roughly the 1976 level by the year 2000. However, within the pensionable population, the number of very old (85 and over) is expected to increase continuously while those aged 75–84 are likely to increase by about 20%. Much the same development is anticipated for Norway and Sweden. Interestingly, in Norway, the number of people aged 60 and over is expected to decrease by about 2% by the year 2000 compared with the 44% increase over the period 1960–1980. The size of the age group 80 years and over, however, is expected to rise by 41% by 2000. Overall, the relative size of the age group 60 and over in Norway is expected

[a] **Hakama, M.** Projection of cancer incidence: experiences and some results in Finland. *World health statistics quarterly*, **33**: 228–240 (1980).

to reach a maximum of 21.2% of the population in 1986. The peak for those aged 80 plus (4.1%) will only be attained after the year 2000.

Projections of the adult population (20–59 years) are also characterized by differential expectations for major subgroups where these have been examined. In Norway, because of the smaller birth cohorts of the 1930s and the early 1940s, the cohorts retiring around the year 2000 will be correspondingly smaller. At the same time, the cohorts entering work will be somewhat larger, with the result that the relative size of this age group is expected to increase from 50% to 56% of the total population by the end of the century. Moreover, the greatest concentration of population within this age group in the future will be at ages 30–49 where economic participation is usually at a maximum. The supply of labour is, therefore, likely to increase and will not decline until the larger cohorts born during the post-war "baby boom" retire.[a]

Conversely, in Hungary, the number of economically active people is expected to decline further during the 1980s. By the latter part of the decade, however, the replacement of labour is expected to improve as the larger, younger cohorts enter working life. By the year 2000, the number of people aged 15–39 is expected to be about 6% larger than in 1980, while those aged 40–49 will have been augmented by about 10%. As the country report notes, the expected increase in the economically active population also depends on other factors: the duration of compulsory education, regulations governing retirement from the workforce, the availability of child care and the adequacy of child care allowances. A further increase in female labour force participation, from 71% to 77%, is also anticipated. Quite the contrary development is expected to occur in Belgium where, after reaching a peak in the 1980s, the number of people in the economically active age groups is projected to decline gradually. In Greece, also, the relative size of the working age population (15–64 years) is expected to decline slightly from 65.1% of the total in 1961 to 62.7% in 2001.

In the report for Great Britain, the population aged 15 years and over was projected only for a 15-year period, thereby avoiding assumptions about the future course of fertility (which is generally more volatile, and consequently more difficult to project, than either mortality or migration). Between 1976, the base year for the projections, and 1991 the population of working age (men aged 15–64, women aged 15–59) was expected to increase by 1.7 million to 34.4 million. Initially, the increase was expected to average about 0.6% per year, slowing progressively throughout the 1980s and then declining by the beginning of the next decade. This basically reflects the changing size of the young cohorts entering the workforce. The population aged 15–19, the ages at which the majority begin economic activity, was projected to increase by 10% between 1976 and 1981 and then to decrease by about one fifth during the 1980s. Overall, by 1991 the size of the age group 45–59

---

[a] Based on fixed labour force participation rates, the size of the labour force is expected to increase by about 8% in the 1980s and by 5% in the 1990s, compared with 2.6% and 1.5% respectively for the total population.

was expected to be about 6% smaller than in 1976, while the population of early middle age (30–44 years) should have grown by about 20% and the number of young adults (15–29) by less than 4%. The number of women of reproductive age was also expected to grow by about 10% over the period because of the larger birth cohorts of 1955–1964 and the fact that women leaving this age group at the end of the decade would be the survivors of the much smaller birth cohorts born immediately prior to and during the earlier part of the Second World War.

Given the degree of uncertainty about the future course of fertility, population projections of the younger age groups must be viewed with added caution. As the Norwegian report notes, projections for that country were based on historically low reproduction rates. The reduction in marriage and fertility rates during the 1970s may well be a temporary phenomenon which could be altered by an active family policy in the future, incorporating more kindergartens and providing greater opportunities for part-time work, especially for mothers. In general, though, the expectation is that there will be relatively fewer young people. According to the Portuguese projections, the ratio of the population aged 65 and over to that aged less than 15 years (an aging indicator) is likely to increase from 0.35 in 1975 to about 0.55 by the year 2000. Moreover, when migration hypotheses are incorporated into the projections, the ratio is projected to rise to almost 0.6 by the end of the century, reflecting the propensity of the young to migrate.

Largely as a consequence of these changes in population structure, the traditional excess of births over deaths is expected to alter in the future. Thus in Sweden, the number of live births is projected to increase gradually to reach a maximum in the early 1990s and to decline thereafter. With population aging continuing meanwhile, the number of deaths is expected to rise with the result that natural increase will cease by 1990, and reach an annual deficit of 11 200 by the year 2000. In the Netherlands, the absolute number of births is expected to increase between 1980 and 1990, mainly because of an expected rise in the number of first births and an increase in the number of marriages. From 1990 onwards, however, a sharp decline in the number of births is anticipated. As in Sweden, the number of deaths will rise progressively and by the turn of the century will exceed the current figure by almost 40%. According to the Hungarian report, the net effect of these two opposite trends will be a reduction of about 400 000 in population size by the year 2000 compared with the present. Moreover, as the Greek study emphasizes, the consequences of population aging extend beyond this immediate impact on vital rates. Specifically, the higher proportion of elderly people is likely to alter the demopathology of the population, with a consequent rise in morbidity from cardiovascular diseases and other chronic conditions.

Finally, it is worthwhile noting that projections of population characteristics other than age structure were attempted in some cases. In Hungary, for example, a more educated population is anticipated, with the proportion of adults who do not complete the obligatory eight grades of primary school projected to decline from 33% at present to 11% by the year 2000. Meanwhile, the proportion who complete secondary school is expected to rise from 23% to 37% by the end of the century, and from 7% to 11% for graduates of tertiary institutions. Not surprisingly, population projections by residential status in Finland indicate that the phenomenon of population aging is likely to be of greater consequence for the urban communes than for rural areas. Between 1980 and 2000, the proportion aged 65 and over is projected to increase from 11.2% to 13.5% in the urban districts, but by only 1.5 percentage points (to 14.7%) in the rural communes. Similarly, the relative decline in the proportion of children aged less than 15 years is likely to be greater in urban centres. In Luxembourg, the decline in the number of Luxembourgeois is expected to continue well into the next century while, concomitantly, the proportion of foreigners is expected to rise to almost a third of the population. The rapid growth of the urban population in Morocco in recent decades is also expected to continue, with over half (58%) of the population likely to be living in urban areas by the turn of the century.

Consequences of demographic change for the health and social services

What are the major health and social implications of these anticipated changes in demographic composition and in the factors that give rise to it? Undoubtedly, population aging is, and will continue to be, one of the principal concerns of those entrusted with the provision of health and social services. As the Norwegian report stresses, the aging of the population carries with it a greater need for nursing homes and other institutions for the elderly. In 1980, for example, there were only about 40 000 beds available in nursing homes and homes for old people in Norway, or about one bed for every ten people aged 70 and over. In addition many of the elderly wish to remain in their own homes or family environment for as long as possible, which will necessitate improved home nursing schemes, better communication facilities and often improvements to the dwellings themselves. Indeed, a 1975 survey found that about 20% of those aged 67 and over who did not live in institutions for the elderly reported that they needed daily help. The greatest need arose among those living in peripheral and inner-city areas. A similar need was also recognized in the Netherlands report as a consequence of increasing emphasis on caring for, rather than attempting to cure, chronic illness among the aged.

With regard to the provision of appropriate health services in anticipation of future developments in morbidity and mortality, the need to focus on specific risk groups becomes paramount. The findings of the Belgian report in this respect are almost certainly indicative of the situation in other countries of the Region. Infant mortality, for example, was found to vary considerably according to socioeconomic and sociocultural characteristics. Migrant groups are especially vulnerable. The higher mortality of adolescents, especially males, from traffic accidents (often related to alcohol abuse) is another area where more effective health education is urgently needed. Adult males in particular would also appear to be especially susceptible to coronary heart disease, for which the major risk factors are reasonably well established. Behaviour modification programmes founded on the results of epidemiological and behavioural research would be a highly desirable component of current and future health strategies aimed at prevention, rather than at costly attempts at cure. It is also recognized that the increase in the number of elderly people, with their characteristic morbidity patterns, will necessitate a corresponding reorientation in the provision of hospitalization and other health services. In this respect, it is encouraging to note that a lead has already been taken by the medical establishment in a number of countries, with the recognition of geriatrics as a specialist medical field.

The immediate implications of the nature and extent of morbidity in the population can be readily assessed from the comprehensive health profile contained in the Netherlands report. According to a 1977 survey only about half the male population and little more than a third of women aged 15 and over considered that they were "healthy". A quarter of them had been, or still were, ill at home in the three-month period preceding the survey, while almost half (45%) had found it necessary to consult a general practitioner. Moreover, one of the ailments most frequently cited for treatment was high blood pressure, a major risk factor for cerebrovascular and coronary heart disease. The number of reported cases of gonorrhoea and syphilis is also rapidly rising, and the same may be assumed true for the vast majority of cases that are not reported. A further 8.5% of the population in 1980 were physically handicapped, largely because of defects of the heart and large vessels and rheumatic conditions. In the same year, over 10% of the population were admitted to hospital, and the admission rate continues to rise. The specific services necessary to treat these patients must continue to anticipate[a] and adapt to the principal causes of hospitalization. For men these are currently diseases of the circulatory system, the respiratory system and the digestive tract, as well as injuries arising from accidents; for women, deliveries and complications associated therewith, as well as diseases of the genitourinary system, account for most admissions. In mental hospitals, where a bimodal age distribution of patients (with peaks at ages 45–54 and 75 years and over) is found, the most common diagnoses are schizophrenia, other psychoses and mental retardation.

The social implications of changes in fertility and family formation patterns are likely to become increasingly pressing in the future. With regard to fertility, adolescent sexual activity is undoubtedly an issue where much greater service provision is necessary, especially in view of the fact that the rapid increase in sexual activity at ever younger ages has not generally been accompanied by a corresponding increase in the use of contraception. In this respect, as the Belgian report notes, adolescents are a vulnerable group requiring special attention, not the least because effective contraceptive behaviour entails a considerable learning process which is particularly difficult at the commencement of sexual activity. Another feature of changing fertility patterns to which attention should be drawn is the considerable

---

[a] A projection of the future demand for the various medical specialties in the light of anticipated changes in the age structure is given in the Netherlands report. According to these estimates, an increase in patient admissions for internal medicine, cardiology, pulmonary medicine, rheumatology, radiology, X-ray diagnosis and radiotherapy can be expected, while a reduction in demand is projected for paediatrics, obstetrics and ear, nose and throat medicine.

reduction in the number and proportion of large families. This has been accompanied by a contraction of the period within marriage during which women engage in childbearing, and a marked reduction in the proportion of women's lives devoted to caring for dependent children. At the same time, community aspirations for higher living standards and more personal motivations have encouraged more and more married women to re-enter the labour force between, or on completion of, childbearing. As a result, there is now a much greater — and indeed urgent — need for more vocational training for women, for improved child care facilities, and for full-time employment conditions that better meet the needs of workers with dependent children. As the Dutch report suggests, the dual role that many married women now increasingly assume has considerable socioeconomic implications — in addition to those for women's health — arising from the division of labour between husband and wife.

One important consequence of the changing age structure of the population, to which little attention has been given, is the rising proportion of men in the population. With falling mortality, the age at which men cease to be in the majority in Great Britain, for example, has risen from 18 years in the late 1940s to about 45 years today. This change in the sex distribution will make it more difficult for men to find marriage partners. The prospects are especially concerning for men born during times of declining births. Since men traditionally look for a bride some years younger than themselves, the pool of women available to these groups of men will be reduced. In fact, this "marriage squeeze" has already resulted in an increase in the marriage rates of women relative to those of men, and the imbalance is likely to worsen in the future unless it can be redressed through selective migration.

A number of changes in demographic phenomena, including smaller families, the desire to leave home at an earlier age, an increase in divorce, greater regional mobility of individuals, and the considerable discrepancy between male and female survival, point to the presence of markedly higher numbers of single people — both young and old — in the future population. The implications of this development for the health and social services are considerable. To begin with, it would appear reasonable to assume that single people will make greater demands on professional services as family support mechanisms become less viable. As the Norwegian study notes, the presence of more single people may lead to a decrease in the number available to care for sick and elderly relatives in their homes. There is, however, as the British report points out, another aspect to this problem of dependency. With the decline in mortality at the older ages, the likelihood of having an elderly relative to care for has increased. At the same time, the middle-aged, who would be called upon to do so, are fewer in number because they belong to smaller birth cohorts. As a result, the period during which a couple have dependent relatives to care for is likely to be longer in future.

The implications of rising divorce rates extend, of course, beyond demographic considerations. Where one or more children were born to the marriage, the parent with custody (normally the mother) will often require day-care facilities for the children, thus increasing the need for kindergartens and other such facilities. Marital dissolution often exposes the children to new or greater psychosocial problems, and these may well necessitate a reorientation of specialized health and social services to cope with them.

As repeatedly emphasized in this chapter, migrants constitute an especially vulnerable group. Moreover, there is a considerable degree of heterogeneity among different ethnic groups in the major immigration countries of the Region, and this must be borne in mind when providing health and social services for them. Common to all population movement, whether internal or external, are the general problems related to integration. These are exacerbated by language difficulties and cultural differences, which often effectively reduce the accessibility and acceptability of health services. Furthermore, given the typical age composition of migrant groups and their generally higher fertility rates compared with the host population, local health and welfare services must be prepared to meet the specific demands for fertility regulation and maternal and child health care.

Many of the implications of an internal move within a country also derive from the age composition of these migrants. As the British report suggests, since these migrants tend to be younger people they are likely to add to the natural increase in the areas in which they settle. Furthermore, outward migration from the inner areas of the major conurbations in the United Kingdom and elsewhere has created a rising demand for educational, housing and ancillary services in the receiving communities. What is perhaps of greater concern, however, is that the younger, more skilled and better qualified people are the ones who leave; the older and less skilled, whose demands on the health and social services (unemployment benefits, etc.) are likely to be somewhat greater, remain behind.

The implications of continued rapid urbanization and population growth in Morocco must also be mentioned here. According to the country report, the growth in employment over the next two decades must average around 3.4% per annum if it is to meet the population requirements in the year 2000 — when 320 000 new jobs will need to be created compared with 115 000 in 1975. By the year 2000, it is also expected that cereal production will satisfy the needs of only about 60% of the population, compared with around 80% in recent years. Furthermore, housing construction has failed to keep pace with the rapid growth of the urban population in the 1970s, resulting in a current deficit of about 700 000 homes; a further 1.1 million dwellings will be required during the 1980s if the projected population growth materializes. At the same time, the level of health infrastructure will need to be increased by around 16% over the period 1980–2000 to provide satisfactory coverage of the health needs of the future population.

In conclusion, it would seem that although the demographic development of countries in the Region over the last two or three decades has differed in some (not unimportant) respects, the issues that must be addressed in the future will for most countries be remarkably similar. Those population subgroups that are especially vulnerable and incur added health risks (migrants, lower socioeconomic classes, adult males) should be the targets of more intensive and effective health education programmes based on admittedly incomplete but nonetheless still substantial evidence about their poorer health profiles. Similarly, the rapidly evolving changes in family formation, in social norms governing behaviour, and in underlying demographic phenomena will continue to alter the social and demographic fabric of society. It is to the needs of these emerging groups, prominent among whom are the elderly, that the health and social services must increasingly be directed. Where, as is often the case, the interrelationship between demographic phenomena and health is poorly understood, more intensive investigation must be pursued in order to provide a more informed basis for future health and social planning.

Part II

Recent demographic trends in the European Region

2

Trends and perspectives in family formation

L. Herberger

The number of families and households (according to United Nations definitions) in a given population is a function of a series of demographic and social factors and of variations in them in the past and future. Of the demographic factors affecting the number of households and families, on the one hand there is the age composition of the population (*inter alia* in terms of family status) and on the other the age at which marriage takes place and the frequency of marriage, as well as the different life expectancies of men and women. The frequency of divorce also plays a part. The frequencies of marriage and of divorce are, for their part, influenced by a multitude of social factors. Investigation of the interaction between demographic and social factors is a very complex matter and will not be dealt with here.

In this chapter, which investigates families and households in Europe, only demographic characteristics will be taken into consideration. In studies of this sort, the point of departure lies in variations in the age–sex composition of the population over a period of time. Findings for the years 1960–1980 are available for this purpose, as well as the population projections drawn up by WHO for the countries of Europe for the period 1980–2000. Data on vital statistics will also be studied, i.e. the mean age of marriage and that of divorce as a function of variations in the age-specific marriage and divorce rates for men and women during the period 1960–1980. Finally, some data on the structure of households will be given. As a consequence, the main emphasis of the study is on the comparison between 1960 and 1980, since demographic trends over the last 20 years can provide indications on future trends and, hence, possible trends in subsequent development.

A number of problems are encountered in undertaking a long-term international comparison of this nature. For example, data for comparable age groups are not always available for all countries in the same years. For the present comparison, therefore, reporting years that are as close as possible to 1960 and to 1980 have been chosen. The age groups used have been compiled so that, as far as possible, they give all the characteristics investigated for uniform age groups. Admittedly, this means that only very crude age groupings have been established.

Data have been drawn principally from publications of the United Nations, in particular the *Demographic yearbook*. The publications of the United Nations Statistical Office for Europe were also used, together with national statistical yearbooks and monographs, where available, produced by European countries for the International Population Year, 1974.

Variations in Family and Population Composition between 1960 and 1980

During the period under consideration population increase varied widely among the different European countries (Tables 1 and 2). Around 1960 the age structure of populations already showed considerable differences in the various European countries. Two basic patterns could be distinguished: (*a*) countries with a large proportion of children and young people (below the age of 15) and a relatively small proportion of the elderly (65 years of age and over) in the total population, and (*b*) countries with a relatively low proportion of children and young people and a relatively high proportion of the elderly.

The trend towards relative aging is in part due to a higher life expectancy, which is more strongly marked among the female than among the male population. In the coming two decades, the population increases in most countries will be felt more weakly than in the previous two decades. If the decrease in births that occurred over the last 20 years, continues into the next two decades, the proportion of children and young people in the total population will be still further reduced, though to a lesser extent in most countries. The relative aging of the population, with its reduction in the proportion of children and young people, will continue — albeit at a slower rate — during the period 1980–2000.

A first departure point in relation to variations in household and family structures is the age group and family composition of the population. In general the proportion of unmarried people in the 45–65-year age group has fallen considerably, the exceptions being Bulgaria, Italy and Spain. The proportion married among those aged 65 or over has risen in all countries except Ireland, where the proportion has fallen among both men and women. The trend in the proportion married in the 15–45-year age group is less clear; the proportion has risen in most countries of Western Europe, with the exception of the Scandinavian countries, and in certain countries in Southern and Eastern Europe.

The proportion of widowed people in most European countries has risen in the age group 65 or over, and the same is true, though to a lesser extent, for divorcees. In general, this holds good for both men and women although in some countries, such as the Netherlands, the proportion of widowers over 65 years of age fell slightly between 1960 and 1970 and that of widows rose. A similar varied picture, at least in general terms, is evident for divorcees in Bulgaria, the German Democratic Republic, Ireland and Switzerland. The

Table 1. Percentage changes in the married and unmarried populations aged 15 years and over in the countries of Europe, in different periods between 1960 and 1980[a]

Country	Change from/to	Unmarried		Married	
		Male	Female	Male	Female
Eastern Europe					
Bulgaria	1965/1975	+ 4.2	- 0.2	+ 8.1	+ 8.3
Czechoslovakia	1961/1970	+17.4	+14.6	+ 7.0	+ 7.2
German Democratic Republic	1966/1978	+32.6	+10.6	- 1.9	- 3.1
Hungary	1960/1976	+11.4	- 2.4	+11.9	+11.5
Romania	1966/1977	+20.2	+25.0	+10.7	+ 9.8
Northern Europe					
Denmark	1960/1980	+35.3	+26.2	+ 6.7	+ 6.9
England & Wales	1961/1978	+15.0	+ 0.2	+ 5.0	+ 4.7
Finland	1960/1979	+29.6	+15.2	+16.5	+16.6
Iceland	1960/1975	+16.0	+ 4.5	+38.7	+34.4
Ireland	1961/1979	+ 8.3	+ 6.9	+36.6	+34.0
Norway	1960/1979	+19.7	+ 9.7	+14.3	+14.0
Sweden	1960/1979	+26.2	+18.1	+ 0.6	+ 0.6
Southern Europe					
Italy	1966/1973	- 0.7	- 3.3	+ 3.7	+ 4.9
Portugal	1960/1973	-21.5	-18.3	+ 6.3	+ 8.1
Spain	1960/1970	+ 3.6	- 0.6	+17.1	+16.3
Western Europe					
Austria	1961/1979	+17.7	+ 2.7	+ 6.1	+ 5.7
Belgium	1961/1970	+ 9.2	+ 3.8	+ 4.5	+ 4.5
France	1962/1978	+17.0	+15.7	+20.2	+17.7
Federal Republic of Germany	1961/1979	+30.1	+ 7.7	+10.1	+10.2
Luxembourg	1960/1970	0	0	+ 3.8	+ 6.4
Netherlands	1960/1979	+36.3	+21.7	+33.7	+33.2
Switzerland	1960/1970	+ 5.6	0	+16.7	+20.0

[a] Excluding Albania, Greece, Malta, Poland, the USSR and Yugoslavia, for which no data are available.

Table 2. Percentage changes in the widowed and divorced populations aged 15 years and over in the countries of Europe, in different periods between 1960 and 1980[a]

Country	Change from/to	Widowed		Divorced	
		Male	Female	Male	Female
Eastern Europe					
Bulgaria	1965/1975	+17.8	+15.3	+ 69.0	+ 61.1
Czechoslovakia	1961/1970	+ 6.5	+11.5	+ 53.7	+ 48.4
German Democratic Republic	1966/1978	- 4.2	- 7.0	+112.5	+ 34.3
Hungary	1960/1976	+18.2	+13.5	+189.6	+117.6
Romania	1966/1977	+49.2	+11.4	+ 91.0	+ 29.4
Northern Europe					
Denmark	1960/1980	+ 4.2	+46.7	+113.7	+ 84.2
England & Wales	1961/1978	+ 2.9	+14.2	+369.5	+261.8
Finland	1960/1979	+ 8.9	+24.3	+196.2	+136.2
Iceland	1960/1975	0	+40.0	+200.0	+100.0
Ireland	1961/1979	- 17.4	+11.9		
Norway	1960/1979	0	+47.4	+210.0	+167.9
Sweden	1960/1979	- 3.3	+41.6	+203.0	+176.4
Southern Europe					
Italy	1966/1973	+ 0.3[b]	+ 4.9[b]		
Portugal	1960/1973	- 8.5	+ 3.7	+ 30.0	+ 26.3
Spain	1960/1970	+ 0.7	+ 5.5	+275.0	+205.9
Western Europe					
Austria	1961/1979	- 4.0	+ 5.3	+ 49.2	+ 41.0
Belgium	1961/1970	- 3.0	+10.7	+ 22.9	+ 18.4
France	1962/1978	- 4.8	+ 7.4	+ 98.7	+ 84.4
Federal Republic of Germany	1961/1979	- 0.5	+14.6	+109.2	+ 54.8
Luxembourg	1960/1970	- 16.7	+16.7	+400.0	+300.0
Netherlands	1960/1979	+ 3.5	+64.2	+238.9	+172.1
Switzerland	1960/1970	0	+15.3	+262.5	+ 80.7

[a] Excluding Albania, Greece, Malta, Poland, the USSR and Yugoslavia, for which no data are available.

[b] Including divorcees.

increase in divorcees in the age group 15–45 years indicates that the proportion of one-parent and one-person households has also increased. A growing number of people are experiencing living in a one-parent or a one-person household.

From the trends shown, a number of conclusions may already be drawn in relation to developments in numbers and patterns of households. The decline in the birth rate results in a reduction in family size; in other words the number of children per family is reduced and the number of childless families is increased. This underlying future trend may be counterbalanced, or its effect may be reduced in the short term, when large cohorts reach marriageable age. In addition, the growing trend towards widowhood and divorce is important in the development of household structure. In the long term, it would lead to a further increase in single-person households.

Marriage and Divorce

Trends in marriage between 1960 and 1980 (Table 3)
Around 1960, the mean age at first marriage for men and women in Southern and Northern Europe was higher than that for Western and Eastern Europe. For example, the mean age at marriage was 28.8 years (Spain) and 27.3 years (Sweden) for men and 26.0 years (Spain) and 24.3 years (Sweden) for women. Conversely, the mean age at marriage was for example 25.8 years (Federal Republic of Germany) and 23.9 years (German Democratic Republic) for men, and 23.4 years (Belgium) and 21.8 years (Bulgaria) for women.

The age difference between men and women at their first marriage was evident in all European countries. In Denmark, Greece, Hungary, Ireland, Italy and Sweden, men were on average three to four years older than their wives at the time of first marriage. In Austria, Belgium, France, the Federal Republic of Germany, the Netherlands, Poland, Portugal, Spain and the United Kingdom the age difference was between two and three years. The age difference in the German Democratic Republic was particularly narrow at 1.4 years. Considerable deviations in age difference between men and women existed within the three subregions of Northern, Eastern and Southern Europe as well. Thus, while the age difference in Greece was four years on average, in Portugal it was 2.1 years. In Western Europe the differences were relatively narrow, varying between 2.2 years in the Federal Republic of Germany and 2.7 years in Austria.

In most European countries, the mean age of marriage has fallen during the period under consideration, particularly in the Netherlands where the reduction was 5.6 years for men and 6.1 years for women. This trend was most homogeneous in Western Europe, and on a similar scale for both men and women. Only in Switzerland has the mean age at marriage, for both men and women, increased. In Eastern Europe the mean age at marriage for men fell in all countries; for women it also fell in the German Democratic Republic, Hungary and Poland but rose slightly in Bulgaria and Czechoslovakia. The trend was less homogeneous in Northern and Southern Europe, but there too a general fall in the mean age of marriage for both men and women was evident.

Table 3. Percentage changes in average age of marriage for the countries of Europe, in different periods between 1960 and 1980

Country	Change from/to	Average age of marriage			
		Total		First marriage	
		Male	Female	Male	Female
Eastern Europe					
Bulgaria	1967/1974	- 1.1	+ 0.4	- 0.4	+ 0.9
Czechoslovakia	1966/1977	- 0.4	+ 2.5	- 0.8	+ 1.4
German Democratic Republic	1960/1978	- 4.0	- 4.8	- 2.5	- 5.3
Hungary	1960/1978	- 6.9	- 3.6	- 6.7	- 3.7
Poland	1962/1975	- 5.7	- 3.6	- 6.1	- 4.2
Romania	1967/1974	- 3.6	- 2.9	- 2.0	0
Northern Europe					
Denmark	1960/1978	+ 6.7	+10.5	+ 4.2	+ 6.6
Finland	1965/1978	+ 4.1	+ 4.5	+ 3.6	+ 4.3
Iceland	1967/1975	- 0.4	+ 1.7	- 1.2	+ 0.4
Ireland	1960/1975	- 12.6	- 9.2	- 12.1	- 8.1
Norway	1960/1978	- 3.8	- 1.6	- 4.8	- 3.7
Sweden	1960/1978	+ 7.2	+ 8.9	+ 4.0	+ 6.2
United Kingdom	1960/1978	+ 3.9	+ 5.5	- 1.9	- 1.7
Southern Europe[a]					
Greece	1960/1977	- 2.8	- 8.1	- 2.8	- 8.2
Italy	1960/1977	- 4.8	- 3.2	- 5.2	- 3.6
Malta	1967/1978	+ 1.5	+ 2.1	+ 0.8	+ 2.1
Portugal	1960/1978	- 0.7	- 2.4	- 4.5	- 4.4
Spain	1960/1975	- 8.2	- 8.4	- 8.3	- 8.4
Yugoslavia	1966/1977	- 1.1	- 1.6	0	+ 0.9
Western Europe					
Austria	1961/1978	- 2.7	- 2.3	- 2.7	- 3.0
Belgium	1960/1977	- 5.4	- 5.6	- 5.4	- 6.0
France	1960/1977	- 4.6	- 3.6	- 4.6	- 3.4
Federal Republic of Germany	1960/1978	+ 1.4	+ 1.2	0	- 2.5
Luxembourg	1966/1975	- 1.1	+ 0.4	- 1.9	- 1.7
Netherlands	1960/1978	- 4.2	- 4.7	- 5.6	- 6.1
Switzerland	1966/1978	+ 2.8	+ 3.8	+ 3.0	+ 3.7
USSR	1966/1975	- 2.6	- 6.0	- 6.2	- 9.6

[a] Excluding Albania, for which no data are available.

Changes in age-specific marriage rates between 1960 and 1980 (Table 4)
The age-specific marriage rate shows the number of people who have married at a given age as a proportion of the total number of men and women of the same age. The variations that took place up to the end of the 1970s are shown on the basis of these rates. Unfortunately, the marriage rates are not related in every country to the same age groups. Similarly, the base age and the length of the period considered do not always correspond. The age-specific marriage rates for men and women, like the mean age at marriage, also show considerable differences. If the marriage rates for men aged between 15 and 30 years are compared, in 20 out of the 26 countries studied the rates range between 40% and 60%. Values of over 60% were reached in the German Democratic Republic, the Federal Republic of Germany, Hungary and Poland, with the German Democratic Republic attaining an exceptional figure (77%). Greece (40%) and Ireland (32%) showed exceptionally low marriage rates.

For women aged between 15 and 30 years, the marriage rate was higher on average than among men of the same age range, since in general women marry earlier than men. For example, in 10 of the 26 countries studied the rates for women aged between 15 and 30 years were 65% or more, with the rate for the German Democratic Republic of 81% being by far the highest. However, marriage among women at these ages in the Federal Republic of Germany was particularly high as well, with a rate of 74%. In most countries the rate was between 50% and 75%, being particularly low in Ireland (44%) and Malta (40%).

In 10 of the 26 European countries, the marriage rates for men aged between 30 and 45 years were relatively high, with values lying between 16% and 33%. If marriage among 30- to 45-year-olds is compared with 15- to 30-year-olds in these countries, two distinct groups may be identified. On the one hand are countries where men generally married relatively late, and which therefore showed relatively high rates for the older group and relatively low rates for the younger group; these include Greece, Ireland, Italy, Norway, Spain and Switzerland. To the other group belong countries where the frequency of marriage was generally high, and which therefore showed high rates among both groups; these included Austria, the Federal Republic of Germany, Hungary and Poland. As a consequence of the higher rate among women than among men in the age group 15–30 years, the rate for women in the age group 30–45 years is lower than that for men.

During the period studied, a fall in marriage rates among men and women of all ages occurred in most European countries, and was particularly marked in the Western European countries. Countries showing a particularly strong decline in marriage rates (between 30% and 51%) were Austria, Denmark, the Federal Republic of Germany, Sweden and Switzerland. Austria, Denmark and the Federal Republic of Germany showed relatively high rates around the year 1960, and in contrast Sweden and Switzerland showed relatively low rates. A considerable increase in rates for men and women aged between 15 and 30 years was also found in Greece, Ireland, Malta and Portugal. There was a relatively low reduction in the marriage rate (between 1% and 19%) among men and women aged

Table 4. Percentage changes in age-related marriage rates for the countries of Europe, in different periods between 1960 and 1980[a]

Country	Change from/to	Males				Females			
		15–29 years	30–44 years	45–54 years	55+ years	15–29 years	30–44 years	45–54 years	55+ years
Eastern Europe									
Bulgaria	1961/1979	+ 1.0	+ 7.3[b]	- 20.5[c]	- 50.0[d]	+ 2.5	- 1.3[b]	- 25.7[c]	- 43.7[d]
Czechoslovakia	1961/1977	+ 4.9	0	+32.4	+10.5	+ 4.9	+16.4	+29.6	+14.3
German Democratic Republic	1964/1979	- 12.1	+ 9.3	- 27.1	- 51.2	- 5.7	- 2.4	- 34.0	- 45.5
Hungary	1960/1979	- 4.5	- 39.6[b]	- 35.2[c]	- 18.9[d]	- 1.4	- 34.9[b]	- 29.7[c]	0[d]
Poland	1960/1979	- 13.1	- 30.9[b]	- 29.3[c]	- 29.3[d]	- 5.4	- 31.1[b]	- 32.6[c]	+13.3[d]
Romania	1964/1979	+ 5.3	- 6.4	- 22.8	- 22.9	+ 7.3	- 17.0	- 7.7	0
Northern Europe									
Denmark	1960/1978	- 42.3	- 2.0	- 2.0	+ 5.0	- 38.5	+24.7	+ 6.3	+28.6
England & Wales	1961/1977	- 16.0	+33.6	+46.3	+ 3.0	- 12.6	+55.4	+36.1	+ 6.3
Finland	1960/1979	- 29.6	- 14.1	- 40.0	- 41.7	- 27.1	- 6.6	- 41.2	- 37.5
Iceland	1961/1977	- 21.4	- 20.1	- 37.7	- 35.0	- 22.4	- 12.1	- 41.0	- 37.5
Ireland	1961/1975	+41.9	- 32.6	- 36.4	- 40.0	+19.6	- 30.5	- 5.9	- 44.4
Norway	1960/1978	- 17.3	- 28.9	- 29.7	- 50.0	- 22.1	- 22.2	- 43.3	- 28.6
Sweden	1960/1979	- 50.5	- 4.5	0	- 28.6	- 46.2	+16.1	- 6.7	- 33.3

Southern Europe									
Greece	1961/1978	+20.1	- 30.2	- 30.2	- 27.3	+15.9	- 37.4	+17.6	+66.7
Italy	1961/1978	- 10.1	- 53.8	- 29.6	- 6.7	- 18.6	- 44.0	0	+40.0
Malta	1962/1979	+18.2	+ 6.3	+39.1	+16.7	+36.8	+48.1	+55.6	0
Portugal	1960/1975	+56.9	- 11.5	+24.4	+39.3	+49.2	- 17.0	+37.9	+70.0
Spain	1960/1977	+13.8	- 50.6	- 52.2	- 45.0	+ 5.4	- 53.0	- 45.2	- 40.0
Yugoslavia	1961/1978	- 14.3	- 26.0	- 35.2	- 10.3	- 11.0	- 34.4	- 13.3	+33.3
Western Europe									
Austria	1960/1979	- 29.5	- 43.6	- 46.5	- 39.5	- 30.4	- 38.6	- 34.1	- 30.0
Belgium	1961/1978	- 15.5	- 45.9	- 28.1[e]	- 50.0[f]	+37.4	+ 2.7	- 20.0[e]	0[f]
France	1962/1978	- 25.4	+ 8.6	- 13.5	- 15.8	- 25.2	+ 4.3	- 13.3	- 22.2
Federal Republic of Germany	1961/1979	- 45.0	- 43.8	- 50.0	- 40.0	- 43.8	- 36.5	- 28.6	- 11.1
Luxembourg	1960/1978	- 25.2	- 27.1	- 6.7		- 28.8	- 22.2	0	
Netherlands	1960/1978	- 27.0	- 40.6	- 24.3	- 38.5	- 28.2	- 30.0	- 36.7	- 36.4
Switzerland	1960/1979	- 31.6	- 26.8	- 40.0	- 50.0	- 32.5	- 27.7	- 41.7	- 50.0

[a] Excluding Albania and the USSR, for which no data are available.

[b] 30-40 years.

[c] 40-50 years.

[d] 50 years and over.

[e] 45-60 years.

[f] 60 years and over.

15–30 years in England & Wales, the German Democratic Republic, Hungary, Italy, Poland and Yugoslavia.

There was a sharp reduction in marriage rates for both men and women aged 30–45 years in 13 of the 26 countries studied, whereas a strikingly high rise in the marriage rate for that age group occurred in England & Wales. Countries where the rate for men aged between 30 and 45 years fell while that of women increased, included Belgium, Denmark and Sweden; the reverse was true in Bulgaria and the German Democratic Republic.

The general trend towards a reduction in marriage rates applied also to men and women over 45 years of age, particularly in Western European countries. In 14 of the 26 countries studied, the reduction in rates for this age group reached partial values of between 25% and 50%. An increase in marriage among men and women over the age of 45 was found in Czechoslovakia, England & Wales, Malta and Portugal.

There is not necessarily a contradiction between a decrease in the mean age of marriage and a diminution in the age-specific marriage rates; it may mean, however, that although the marriage curve is falling off, those who marry are marrying somewhat earlier. With regard to trends in the numbers and structure of families and households this means that, irrespective of whether children are born into families or not, families are starting younger. The fall-off in marriage and the increase of the number of single-person households among younger age groups probably indicates a similar social evolution.

Trends in the mean age at divorce between 1960 and 1980 (Table 5)
The trends occurring up to the end of the 1970s are based on figures beginning in about 1966. The rates of change shown should again be considered in the light of the fact that they relate partially to different juridical and social situations. Both the average age at divorce and the divorce rates are affected by the particular content of the divorce laws in effect and by cultural, in particular religious, considerations. These varying facts considerably reduced the possibility of comparing the available data.

Because women marry on average between two and four years earlier than men, the age at divorce among women is correspondingly lower. Of a total of 23 European countries, in 16 the average age for men was 36–39 years, and in 17 countries that for women was 33–36 years. A relatively high age at divorce was displayed by men in Portugal (43 years) and Italy (51 years), the mean age at divorce among women in Portugal being 40 years, in Poland 42 years and in Italy 48 years. The relatively high age at divorce is directly linked with the relatively high age at marriage in these countries. Countries with particularly low ages at divorce among men included Albania and, among women, Albania, Hungary and Romania.

During the period under review, the age at divorce among men fell in 14 countries, rose in seven and remained unchanged — compared with the situation in 1966 — in two countries, Poland and Yugoslavia. In 16 European countries the age at divorce among women fell, and rose in seven countries. As a rule, the trend was in the same direction for both sexes. In Poland and Yugoslavia, however, the age of divorce among women fell

Table 5. Percentage changes in the mean age at divorce for the countries of Europe, in different periods between 1960 and 1980[a]

Country	Change from/to	Males	Females
Eastern Europe			
Bulgaria	1966/1979	- 1.9	- 1.8
Czechoslovakia	1966/1978	- 4.3	- 3.5
German Democratic Republic	1966/1979	- 2.0	- 2.4
Hungary	1968/1979	- 3.0	- 1.8
Poland	1966/1976	0	- 15.6
Romania	1966/1974	+ 6.7	+ 7.1
Northern Europe			
Denmark	1966/1979	+ 0.8	+ 1.7
England & Wales	1966/1979	- 2.1	- 1.4
Finland	1966/1978	- 7.4	- 8.3
Iceland	1966/1975	- 8.0	- 6.6
Norway	1966/1978	- 2.8	- 3.3
Sweden	1966/1979	+ 1.1	+ 2.3
Southern Europe			
Albania	1960/1964	+ 0.6	- 0.7
Italy	1971/1973	- 7.2	- 7.3
Portugal	1966/1975	+ 1.2	+ 1.3
Yugoslavia	1966/1977	0	- 0.3
Western Europe			
Austria	1966/1979	+ 3.1	+ 3.9
Belgium	1966/1975	- 2.8	- 3.0
France	1966/1977	- 7.5	- 7.0
Federal Republic of Germany	1966/1979	+ 1.3	+ 2.6
Luxembourg	1966/1979	- 3.9	- 1.4
Netherlands	1965/1979	- 3.1	- 2.2
Switzerland	1966/1979	- 3.0	- 2.5

[a] Excluding Greece, Ireland, Malta, Spain and the USSR, for which no data are available.

while it remained relatively unchanged among men; the rates of change here were generally relatively low. The reduction in the age at divorce among men ranged between 2% and 8% and among women between 1% and 16%. In countries where the age at divorce has been rising the increase for men and women varied between 1% and 7%.

Changes in age-specific divorce rates between 1960 and 1980 (Table 6)
Age-specific divorce rates show the number of men or women of a given age who have divorced during a given period as a proportion of all married men or women of the same age. International comparison of age-specific divorce rates, and the changes thereto, is difficult because the period investigated is of different length for different countries: the first and last years given are not always the same. In addition, as mentioned above, it should be remembered that the divorce rates are affected by the characteristics of the divorce laws as well as by cultural considerations, particularly those of a religious nature. These different basic facts considerably reduce the comparability of the figures given from one country to another, though not comparisons over time for a given country.

In 1960, age-specific divorce rates in the four subregions of Europe displayed considerable differences. As a rule, the lowest were to be found in Southern Europe and the highest in Eastern Europe, though for Southern Europe data are available only for Greece, Italy and Portugal. In these three countries, the age-specific divorce rates were generally lower than 2% and often below 1%. In Eastern Europe, nearly all age-specific divorce rates were greater than 2% (except for age groups over 55 years) and, among the age groups between 20 and 45 years, the values varied between 2% and 11%. In Northern Europe, divorce rates in the same age groups reached on average lower values than in Eastern Europe: between 2% and 8%. Generally speaking, in the countries of Western Europe the rates were considerably lower than in Northern and Eastern Europe, reaching values between 2% and 5%.

In almost all European countries, age-specific divorce rates rose during the period studied, the tendency being particularly noticeable in Western Europe. Thus, the divorce rate for men aged between 20 and 30 years practically doubled in Switzerland, almost tripled in Belgium, France and the Netherlands, and even quadrupled in Luxembourg. The increase for women of the same age range in these countries was not so great. Among men and women in the higher age groups too, the divorce rate has been rising noticeably in the countries of Europe.

Within this general picture, it is noticeable that the countries with particularly marked increases in their divorce rates were primarily those which, in 1960, displayed relatively low divorce rates. The link between the two facts is particularly striking among the Western European countries mentioned above and in Southern Europe. The reverse is true for the Eastern European countries, where, on average, the highest divorce rates were found at the beginning of the period under consideration, particularly in the German Democratic Republic, Hungary and Romania. Romania is the only country in Europe in which the divorce rates among men and women have fallen for all age groups. In Europe as a whole, there has been a tendency for age-related divorce rates to level off in relation to one another. This may indicate that the changes in divorce behaviour started at different points in time, and that these changes proceeded in different ways. It seems, however, that — with respect to the pattern of divorce behaviour — a fairly uniform situation has now been reached in Europe.

In terms of family and household numbers and patterns, the basic result of divorce is more and more one-parent and single-person households, with more and more people experiencing a change of household during their life. The possibility of remarriage must also be borne in mind, so that dissolution of marriage may lead to the formation of new families and households. Naturally, the same is also true for marriages that end with the death of one of the partners. The probability of remarriage depends on the age and sex of the surviving partner. All other circumstances being equal, rising divorce rates, accompanied by lower age at divorce, mean that the probability of remarriage and the possibility for the reconstitution of a family have increased.

Households

At the beginning of the 1960s, in 20 of the 24 countries in Europe for which figures are available, the mean size of households ranged between three and four people. In Denmark, the German Democratic Republic, the Federal Republic of Germany and Sweden there were on average fewer than three people per household, while in Malta there were, conversely, more than four. In 12 of these 20 countries, the proportion of one- and two-person households was higher than 40%. Particularly high figures for single- and two-person households were encountered in the German Democratic Republic (58%), Denmark and Sweden (49%), Belgium (48%), Austria, France and the Federal Republic of Germany (47%) and Great Britain (46%). In 8 out of 22 European countries, households with five or more people amounted to a quarter or more of all households. Higher than average figures for large households were encountered in Malta (37%), Ireland (36%), Yugoslavia (35%) and Portugal (32%).

Changes in household structure between 1960 and 1980 (Table 7)
With the exception of the German Democratic Republic, the number of households increased in all European countries during the period under consideration. For countries with an approximately 20-year observation period, this increase ranged between 15% (Austria) and 50% (Netherlands) while, in countries with an approximately 10-year observation period, the increase ranged between 5% (Portugal) and 30% (Switzerland).

Examining the alterations in the structure of households in countries with an observation period of some 20 years, it can be seen that single-person households had the greatest growth rates, especially in those countries with a comparatively high proportion of one- and two-person households at the beginning of the 1960s (Federal Republic of Germany +46% and +7% respectively; Netherlands +45% and +23% respectively). Countries displaying

Table 6. Percentage changes in age-related divorce rates for the countries of Europe, in different periods between 1960 and 1980[a]

Country	Change from/to	Males				Females			
		20–29 years	30–44 years	45–54 years	55+ years	20–29 years	30–44 years	45–54 years	55+ years
Eastern Europe									
Bulgaria	1961/1979	+ 34.6	+ 54.3[b]	+ 22.2[c]	- 23.1[d]	+ 36.1	+ 48.7[b]	+ 25.0[c]	- 14.3[d]
Czechoslovakia	1961/1978	+100.0	+ 63.5	+ 51.4	+ 40.0	+ 83.8	+ 63.6	+ 63.6	+ 50.0
German Democratic Republic	1964/1979	+ 30.0[e]	+ 70.0	+ 17.9	- 28.6	+ 44.8[e]	+ 92.5	+ 29.2	- 33.3
Hungary	1960/1979	+ 66.7	+ 45.9[b]	+ 35.1[c]	+ 13.0[d]	+ 65.2	+ 57.4[b]	+ 42.5[c]	0[d]
Poland	1960/1976	+ 50.0	+130.8[b]	+115.8[c]	+ 87.5[d]	+ 78.6	+160.0[b]	+153.8[c]	+100.0[d]
Romania	1964/1974	- 70.7	- 37.8	- 47.1	- 95.0	- 54.0	- 40.3	- 38.1	- 60.0
Northern Europe									
Denmark	1960/1978	+ 28.1	+ 83.3	+ 63.4	+ 64.3	+ 40.5	+ 95.3	+ 66.7	+ 57.1
England & Wales	1961/1977	+525.0	+369.0	+355.6[f]	+314.3[d]	+411.1	+374.1	+346.7[f]	+325.0[d]
Finland	1960/1979	+ 87.1	+156.1	+106.9	+ 88.9	+115.0	+170.3	+109.5	+ 80.0
Iceland	1961/1975	+128.9	+ 82.7	+116.7	- 20.0	+ 89.3	+126.2	+ 86.7	- 50.0
Norway	1960/1978	+117.4	+174.2	+125.0	+ 42.9	+116.7	+170.0	+ 93.8	+ 25.0
Sweden	1960/1979	+ 40.5	+110.2	+142.9	+ 90.0	+ 48.3	+131.6	+125.0	+100.0

Southern Europe									
Greece	1969/1975	+ 0.2	+400.0	+100.0	- 10.8	+ 0.5	+300.0	0	- 12.5
Italy	1971/1973	+100.0	+100.0[e]	0[c]	- 23.1[d]	+150.0	+ 44.4[b]	- 5.9[c]	- 25.0[d]
Portugal	1960/1975	+300.0	+100.0	+ 40.0	+100.0	+150.0	+ 75.0	+ 50.0	+100.0
Western Europe									
Austria	1960/1979	+ 53.2	+ 37.5	+ 8.6	+ 66.7	+ 55.2	+ 51.0	+ 25.0	+166.7
Belgium	1961/1978	+207.1	+183.9[g]	+139.1[h]	+150.0[d]	+170.8	+174.2[g]	+135.0[h]	+166.7[d]
France	1962/1977	+214.3	+ 84.8	+ 40.0	+ 50.0	+152.0	+ 80.6	+ 40.0	+ 66.7
Federal Republic of Germany	1961/1979	+ 76.7	+ 23.4	+ 7.7	+ 25.0	+ 80.0	+ 37.8	+ 33.3	+ 66.7
Luxembourg	1960/1978	+336.4	+220.0	+ 55.6		+310.0	+183.3	+ 60.0	
Netherlands	1960/1978	+230.8	+185.2[b]	+159.1[c]	+211.1[d]	+200.0	+200.0[b]	+172.2[c]	+216.7[d]
Switzerland	1960/1979	+123.8	+ 95.6	+ 57.1	+ 37.5	+102.9	+ 95.2	+ 36.4	+ 25.0

[a] Excluding Albania, Ireland, Malta, Spain and the USSR, for which no data are available.

[b] 30–40 years.

[c] 40–50 years.

[d] 50 years and over.

[e] As from 18 years.

[f] 45–50 years.

[g] 30–35 years.

[h] 35–50 years.

Table 7. Percentage changes in household structure in the countries of Europe, in different periods between 1960 and 1980[a]

Country	Change from/to	Private households							Persons	
		Total	Number of persons						Total	Per household
			1	2	3	4	5	6 and more		
Countries with an observation period of some 10 years										
Czechoslovakia	1961/1970	+ 5.4	+26.1	- 12.3	- 5.9	+ 3.5	- 1.0	+ 2.9	+ 4.5	0
Denmark	1965/1970	+11.2							+ 3.8	- 7.1
England & Wales	1966/1971	+ 7.5	+18.2	+ 4.2	- 9.9	- 4.5	- 6.9	- 10.8	- 1.0	- 3.3
Finland	1960/1970	+15.5	+11.2	+13.9	+ 7.9	+ 3.7	- 13.9	- 38.7	+ 3.3	- 9.1
German Democratic Republic	1964/1971	- 3.5	- 4.4	- 8.7	0	+15.6	+17.0	+29.4	+ 1.5	+ 4.0
Greece	1961/1971	+19.3							+ 4.3	- 13.2
Hungary	1960/1970	+ 9.7	+20.7	- 1.9	+ 0.8	+ 1.6	- 13.3	- 23.6	+ 4.7	- 3.2
Ireland	1961/1971	+ 5.7	+ 8.5	+ 1.5	- 4.8	0	+ 0.9	- 2.9	+ 3.8	- 2.5
Italy	1961/1971	+16.3	+20.6	+12.2	0	+ 4.4	- 6.3	- 32.6	+ 7.2	- 8.3

Luxembourg	1960/1970	+12.5	+36.5	+ 0.4	- 10.9	0	- 6.0	- 11.5		- 3.0
Malta	1957/1967	0	+ 8.0	+ 1.0	0	+ 8.7	- 6.8		- 5.0	- 2.4
Portugal	1960/1970	+ 5.0	+20.5	+17.1	+ 1.4	- 1.1	- 10.2	- 18.9	- 1.9	- 5.1
Spain	1960/1970	+17.3							+13.2	- 5.0
Switzerland	1960/1970	+29.8							+16.3	- 12.1
USSR	1959/1970	+16.6							+16.4	0
Yugoslavia	1961/1971	+15.6	- 5.1	+ 5.8	+10.5	+14.5	- 5.8	- 18.1	+10.6	- 5.0
Countries with an observation period of some 20 years										
Austria	1961/1979	+15.3	+31.6	- 0.7	- 16.3	+ 2.7	- 17.1		+ 6.3	- 6.7
Belgium	1961/1977	+ 9.3	- 6.5	+ 2.6	+ 1.4	+13.7	0	- 24.4	+ 8.0	0
France	1962/1975	+21.6	+13.3	+ 3.3	+ 2.7	+ 4.8	- 12.8	- 32.7	+12.9	- 6.5
Federal Republic of Germany	1961/1979	+25.8	+45.6	+ 7.5	- 21.7	- 8.7	- 35.7		+ 9.1	- 13.8
Netherlands	1960/1977	+50.0	+45.2	+22.7	- 11.6	+16.8	- 21.1	- 63.2	+15.8	- 22.2
Norway	1960/1976	+34.5	+94.4	- 5.1	- 23.7	- 24.2	- 25.7	- 44.9	+ 9.9	- 19.4
Poland	1960/1978	+31.3	+ 8.1	+17.3	+20.5	+ 7.1	- 36.5			- 11.4
Sweden	1960/1975	+25.7	+37.0	+15.8	- 21.4	- 12.2	- 32.9	- 63.3	+ 7.6	- 14.3

[a] Excluding Albania, Bulgaria, Iceland and Romania, for which no data are available.

growth rates among three- and four-person households included Austria, Belgium, France and Poland. In all countries with a 20-year observation period, the proportion of large households with five or more persons decreased, this fall being particularly marked in the Netherlands, Norway and Sweden. These countries already had relatively small numbers of large households at the beginning of the observation period.

Above-average growth rates can also be found in countries followed over a 10-year period, particularly among single-person households. These included Luxembourg (+37%), Czechoslovakia (+26%) and Hungary, Italy and Portugal (+21%). At the beginning of the period the proportion of one-and two-person households was relatively low in Italy (30%) and in Portugal (27%), and around the average in Czechoslovakia, Hungary and Luxembourg (about 40%). Countries that showed growth rates not only among one- and two-person households but also among three- and four-person households, even though these were to some extent lower, included Czechoslovakia, Finland, the German Democratic Republic, Hungary, Italy, Malta, Portugal and Yugoslavia. In this last group of countries a shift may have taken place from large households to those of average size. It should be noted that the rates of change given for the German Democratic Republic cover a comparatively small period — 1964–1971. It is nonetheless noteworthy that the German Democratic Republic was the only country where the proportion of one- and two-person households fell while the number of households with five or more persons rose. An increase in the proportion of large households, albeit to a lesser extent, was also found in Czechoslovakia, while everywhere else this proportion fell considerably.

Past Developments and Possible Future Trends (Tables 8 and 9)

It is imperative for all countries, irrespective of whether their own birth rates continue to rise or not, to take note of the alterations that will occur in the age structure of the population as a result of the reduction in the number of births. Today's low birth figures mean tomorrow's low school intakes and subsequently a smaller actively employed population. Over a period of time, these changes may lead to a numerical and qualitative change in the dependency ratio, since this ratio will gradually rise with the so-called aging of the population. As a result of this, efforts must be made to establish what this implies for trends in the numbers and structure of families and households — in other words the social consequences and impact on the health services that may result.

Based on the developments outlined above, a number of theses can be developed about the impact of demographic changes on the health services. Within the scope of these statements, some obvious policy measures can be postulated.

1. From the observations made so far, the reduction in the number of births leads — given no change in the frequency of marriage and divorce — first and foremost to a reduction in the number of children per family and also to a probable increase in the number of childless families. In medical

terms, this shifts the main demand for medical services from maternal and child care to care for the elderly, provided there is no increase in maternal and child care services (e.g. through even greater efforts to reduce maternal and infant mortality). A possible trend of this sort must be seen in connection with the fact that, all things being equal, the growing number of the elderly will mean that additional capacity will be required for their medical care and their needs for social welfare. The scale of the increase in capacity required for the rising numbers of elderly alone must also take into account whether the demand for medical services on the part of the older generations increases or declines. In addition, it must be noted that the break-up of the three-generation household and the declining number of children in families, combined with the increasing number of childless families, mean that social welfare of the elderly will be less frequently provided by the family than before. The increased pressure on the medical services, and in particular on the social services, resulting from this trend may be aggravated still further if the rate of marriage continues to fall. This would imply a reduction in the number of families but not in the number of households. However, it remains to be seen whether this means a reduction in the number of single-person households or in the number of multi-person households. In a multi-generation household, the preventive care and other care for the elderly can be supplied by the younger members of the household. The decline of this household type has induced a shift in the responsibility for (medical) attendance from the family to medical and other institutions.

2. Further consideration should be given to the possible consequence of increased divorce rates. In purely quantitative terms, these trends imply that during their lifetime more people than before establish more than one family. This may impose an additional burden on the medicosocial services. Early divorce without subsequent remarriage will have consequences for the social and health services, similar to those resulting from the reduction in the rate of marriage.

Every transition from one family type to another involves a time of personal crisis with an increased risk of psychological illness. This results in a need for medicosocial care at these times, since people with an unstable family life are less able to help themselves. Also, the intricacies of changing family life mean there is less time available for looking after one's health.

3. Because there is nobody else at home to provide care when necessary, the increasing number of single-person households (both of elderly and younger people) will lead to poorer health care. Also, the time between falling ill and the provision of professional care is likely to increase. For these reasons the organized health services will have to pay more attention to people in these circumstances.

Table 8. Percentage changes in the age pyramid for the countries of Europe, in different periods between 1950 and 1980

Country	Change from/to	Population						
		Total	Males			Females		
			<15 years	15-65 years	65+ years	<15 years	15-65 years	65+ years
Eastern Europe								
Bulgaria	1962/1979	+10.4	- 12.3	- 0.9	+54.3	- 13.7	- 0.8	+44.3
Czechoslovakia	1961/1979	+11.2	- 10.9	+ 0.2	+41.1	- 11.2	- 2.5	+43.7
German Democratic Republic	1960/1979	- 2.6	- 10.3	+ 3.6	+ 1.7	- 4.2	- 5.6	+29.6
Hungary	1960/1979	+ 7.5	- 14.5	+ 0.8	+43.6	- 14.6	- 2.9	+54.0
Poland	1960/1979	+20.4	- 29.9	+12.3	+68.8	- 27.4	+ 5.9	+69.4
Romania	1960/1979	+19.8	- 7.1	- 1.8	+53.4	- 5.6	- 3.2	+43.8
Northern Europe								
Denmark	1960/1979	+11.7	- 15.4	+ 2.5	+24.2	- 16.0	- 1.6	+43.0
England & Wales	1960/1979	+ 6.5	- 7.7	- 0.8	+26.9	- 7.3	- 3.4	+25.9
Finland	1960/1980	+ 7.7	- 33.2	+12.0	+53.4	- 33.3	+ 5.8	+64.4
Iceland	1960/1979	+28.4	- 21.6	+10.9	+20.5	- 20.8	+ 9.1	+20.9
Ireland	1961/1977	+13.3	+ 0.6	+ 0.9	- 6.7	0	- 0.2	+ 0.8
Norway	1960/1979	+13.6	- 13.2	+ 1.3	+24.8	- 13.9	- 1.8	+36.9
Sweden	1960/1979	+10.8	- 9.7	- 1.4	+29.1	- 10.7	- 4.3	+39.2

Southern Europe								
Albania	1950/1975	+98.9	+ 2.0	+ 1.1	- 26.3	+ 5.3	+ 0.7	- 32.9
Greece	1961/1979	+12.6	- 13.5	- 1.4	+65.3	- 13.4	- 2.6	+56.0
Italy	1961/1979	+12.6	- 8.6	- 1.4	+39.0	- 9.8	- 3.2	+41.7
Malta	1960/1979	- 4.3	- 33.8	+23.4	+ 8.8	- 33.8	+17.1	+22.4
Portugal	1960/1980	+12.1	- 7.7	+ 0.6	+31.8	- 10.5	+ 0.5	+28.3
Spain	1960/1977	+20.4	- 2.8	- 1.7	+25.4	- 1.9	- 3.4	+26.8
Yugoslavia	1961/1980	+20.2	- 20.9	+ 7.1	+45.3	- 19.9	+ 4.4	+41.7
Western Europe								
Austria	1961/1979	+ 6.1	- 6.9	- 0.2	+17.6	- 4.9	- 5.2	+31.7
Belgium	1961/1979	+ 7.1	- 13.3	+ 3.4	+ 9.4	- 13.2	0	+21.0
France	1968/1980	+ 2.4	- 6.9	+ 1.9	+ 3.8	- 6.6	+ 1.8	+ 3.1
Federal Republic of Germany	1961/1979	+ 9.8	- 15.7	+ 1.7	+26.9	- 12.6	- 6.3	+54.5
Luxembourg	1960/1978	+14.9	- 7.7	+ 0.4	+13.5	- 9.2	- 2.7	+30.0
Netherlands	1960/1978	+22.0	- 24.4	+10.6	+16.0	- 24.5	+ 5.4	+42.4
Switzerland	1960/1979	+16.3	- 15.1	+ 1.5	+31.0	- 16.8	- 0.8	+37.6
USSR	1959/1975	+21.8	- 11.7	+ 3.8	+31.1	- 7.4	- 2.9	+49.4

Table 9. Possible percentage trends in age for the countries of Europe, in different periods between 1975 and 2000

Country	Change from/to	Population						
		Total	Males			Females		
			<15 years	15-65 years	65+ years	<15 years	15-65 years	65+ years
Eastern Europe								
Bulgaria	1979/2000	+ 9.6	- 7.0	- 2.0	+27.8	- 7.9	- 4.4	+36.2
Czechoslovakia	1979/2000	+12.6	- 7.5	+ 2.6	+ 1.9	- 4.8	+ 2.3	- 2.0
German Democratic Republic	1979/2000	0	-17.0	+ 6.7	- 6.9	- 9.9	+ 6.0	- 9.6
Hungary	1979/2000	+ 5.1	- 8.3	+ 1.2	+ 9.8	- 5.4	- 0.5	+ 9.1
Poland	1979/2000	+16.4	-11.9	+ 1.8	+23.5	-10.0	+ 0.6	+15.6
Romania	1979/2000	+16.7	-13.2	+ 2.4	+24.7	-12.2	+ 0.2	+26.1
Northern Europe								
Denmark	1979/2000	+ 3.3	- 6.4	+ 1.8	+ 1.6	- 5.9	- 1.7	+ 1.8
Finland	1980/2000	+ 6.8	- 3.3	- 1.0	+15.7	- 1.6	- 0.9	+ 6.8
Iceland	1979/2000	+22.6	-17.6	+ 5.9	+14.8	-19.6	+ 6.3	+11.8
Ireland	1977/2000	+25.6	-19.1	+13.2	-16.3	-19.6	+12.0	- 7.6
Norway	1979/2000	+ 8.0	- 6.9	+ 3.1	- 2.4	- 6.0	+ 2.6	- 1.8
Sweden	1979/2000	+ 2.5	- 2.0	+ 1.4	- 3.5	- 2.1	+ 1.0	- 1.1
United Kingdom	1979/2000	+ 1.3	- 7.5	+ 0.8	+ 9.3	- 3.9	+ 2.4	- 3.4

Southern Europe								
Albania	1975/2000	+61.4	- 30.1	+19.4	+35.7	- 30.0	+17.7	+36.7
Greece	1979/2000	+10.0	- 3.0	- 0.3	+20.2	- 5.9	- 4.1	+27.5
Italy	1979/2000	+ 7.1	- 13.2	+ 0.5	+24.6	- 10.8	- 1.4	+20.3
Malta	1979/2000	+22.9	- 17.7	+ 2.9	+37.8	- 14.1	- 2.9	+55.9
Portugal	1980/2000	+15.1	- 15.0	+ 5.6	+ 9.2	- 11.8	+ 1.1	+18.6
Spain	1977/2000	+18.5	- 18.9	+ 2.7	+40.4	- 16.9	+ 1.1	+30.1
Yugoslavia	1980/2000	+15.0	- 15.5	+ 1.2	+41.6	- 15.1	- 1.7	+46.1
Western Europe								
Austria	1979/2000	+ 1.5	- 10.5	+ 4.0	- 1.7	- 4.1	+ 3.6	- 7.5
Belgium	1979/2000	+ 9.4	- 2.3	- 0.1	+ 6.0	+ 1.0	+ 0.3	- 1.8
France	1980/2000	+12.7	- 6.5	+ 1.2	+ 7.3	- 5.7	+ 2.1	- 0.6
Federal Republic of Germany	1979/2000	- 3.1	- 0.5	- 0.3	+ 3.4	+ 1.7	+ 0.3	- 2.1
Luxembourg	1978/2000	- 0.3	- 10.3	- 2.0	+32.1	- 5.9	- 2.1	+16.0
Netherlands	1978/2000	+10.7	- 12.1	+ 2.1	+16.0	- 12.4	+ 1.4	+15.3
Switzerland	1979/2000	+ 2.0	- 5.8	- 1.5	+18.4	- 4.8	- 3.2	+11.8
USSR	1975/2000	+22.6	- 12.8	+ 1.2	+49.2	- 5.9	- 3.2	+30.4

3

Trends and perspectives in fertility

A. Klinger

During the nineteenth century European countries began the process of demographic transition characterized by an improvement in mortality and a decline in fertility. There is considerable variation in the date of this transition in the individual countries. With regard to the changes in fertility, the initiation of the decline spanned nearly a hundred years, based on the median date for attaining a 10% decline in marital fertility during any one decade. The earliest date refers to France (1836) and the latest to Ireland (1928); this process began even later in Albania. In most European countries the decline started between 1890 and 1915; it began earlier only in France, Hungary and Switzerland, and later only in Albania, Ireland, Italy, Portugal and the USSR.

In general, the decline in fertility was more or less continuous, with only the First World War interrupting the process. In most of the belligerent countries, the substantial decline in births during the war years was followed by a significant increase for a short period immediately afterwards. By the second half of the 1930s in most European countries fertility was not even sufficient for replacement, and in the period prior to the Second World War zero population growth became widespread in Europe.

In the period following the Second World War, European fertility developed in different directions. In one group of countries — consisting mainly of the countries of Northern and Western Europe — a new trend could be observed: the number of births increased steadily compared with the very low level of the pre-war period. Indeed, for a period of about 20 years the decline stopped and a higher fertility level prevailed. This was the period of the "baby boom", which lasted until about 1965 and was followed first by a slow and later, especially in the second half of the 1970s, by a more and more rapid decline in fertility. Consequently, in almost all countries fertility fell well under the replacement level. This phase now seems to have come to an end, and in some countries fertility has begun to increase again in recent years. Some demographers in fact view this as a sign of a possible recovery, which might become the fifth phase of the demographic transition for this group of countries (*1*).

The development has been quite different in most countries of Southern Europe. Here the change was less apparent after the Second World War. Fertility was relatively high and decreased slowly until the end of the 1970s. Only then did the decrease become more intensive. As a result, in these countries one can only speak of one phase in the process of fertility decline, and this has yet to fall below replacement level.

The fertility of the countries of Eastern Europe developed in yet another direction. Here the number of births scarcely increased or rose only for a very short period after the Second World War. From the 1950s on, the decline in births became more distinct and lasted until the middle of the 1960s. After this — partly because of the impact of population policy measures — fertility ceased to decline and the number of births even increased. Thus in these countries the sub-replacement fertility of the 1960s was followed by a positive fertility level which may, of course, decline again. The development of fertility in the USSR was similar. In this case, however, the decrease began from a high level and was slower; also, the present increase is further from the level of zero growth.

The fertility situation of the three other countries of the Region — Algeria, Morocco and Turkey — is quite different from that of the European countries. None of these nations has yet attained the phase of demographic transition. In all three countries, birth rates are still very high and the estimated decline in recent years has been quite small.

Trends in Crude Birth Rates

In this section the trends of the last two decades will be described in greater detail. To begin with, the present levels and changes in fertility are examined on the basis of crude live-birth rates given in Table 1. In the five-year period 1975–1979 there was great variation in the number of live births per 1000 population in the European Region. In Western Europe, crude birth rates are lower by one quarter and in Northern Europe by over one fifth compared with the overall average. Southern Europe is around the average for Europe. The difference between the maximum (USSR) and minimum (Western Europe) amounts to 6.5 births per 1000, i.e. a difference of 55%.

The differences were still quite pronounced during 1960–1964. The highest rate was still found in the USSR, although the rate was lowest in Eastern Europe as a whole compared with other regions. Birth rates were higher in Northern and Western Europe and even more so in Southern Europe. The major shift in the level of fertility was caused by the different developments in the individual regions. Between 1960–1964 and 1975–1979, the birth rate remained constant only in Eastern Europe; in all the other regions it decreased.

The changes in the regions were not, of course, uniform in the countries of those regions. Similarly, birth rates based on regional averages were not uniform either. Various groups of countries can therefore be identified on the basis of the trend in live-birth rates over the last 20 years.

Table 1. Crude live-birth rates in the European Region, 1950–2000[a]

Region and country	1950–1954	1960–1964	1975–1979	1985–1989	1995–1999
Eastern Europe					
Bulgaria	21.7	16.9	16.2	14.6	14.2
Czechoslovakia	22.0	16.3	18.3	15.2	15.4
German Democratic Republic	16.1	17.4	13.1	12.8	11.2
Hungary	21.1	13.6	16.0	12.7	12.7
Poland	30.1	20.1	19.2	16.5	14.6
Romania	24.9	16.7	18.8	16.8	16.3
Total	23.6	17.5	17.5	15.3	14.4
Northern Europe					
Denmark	17.9	17.0	12.5	12.0	12.0
Finland	22.8	18.1	13.6	12.2	11.0
Iceland	27.9	26.1	18.3	16.3	14.7
Ireland	21.4	21.8	21.6	20.3	19.1
Norway	18.7	17.4	12.9	13.1	13.0
Sweden	15.5	14.5	11.5	10.2	11.2
United Kingdom	15.9	18.2	12.0	12.5	12.7
Total	16.7	17.9	12.5	12.6	12.4
Southern Europe					
Albania	38.2	38.9	30.3	24.8	19.2
Greece	10.4	18.1	15.6	15.9	15.1
Italy	18.3	18.8	13.3	12.7	11.8
Malta	29.3	22.6	17.9	15.9	13.8
Portugal	24.1	24.0	18.2	16.9	15.2
Spain	20.3	21.5	17.9	16.5	15.6
Yugoslavia	28.8	22.1	17.7	15.2	13.8
Total	21.2	20.7	16.1	14.9	13.8
Western Europe					
Austria	15.0	18.5	11.5	12.3	11.5
Belgium	16.7	17.1	12.4	12.4	11.8
France	19.5	18.0	13.8	13.4	12.7
Federal Republic of Germany	15.8	18.0	9.8	11.2	10.9
Luxembourg	14.7	16.0	11.1	10.7	9.9
Netherlands	22.1	20.9	12.6	12.6	12.4
Switzerland	17.3	18.5	11.6	11.0	10.6
Total	17.6	18.2	11.8	12.2	11.8
Europe (except USSR)	19.8	18.7	14.4	13.8	13.1
USSR	26.3	22.3	18.3	18.1	16.4
Europe total	21.8	19.9	15.8	15.3	14.3
Algeria	51.0	50.4	47.5	45.6	35.7
Morocco	50.4	50.1	45.4	40.8	31.9
Turkey	44.9	41.0	34.9	31.3	23.8

[a] Five-year averages. Projections based on United Nations medium variant as assessed in 1980.

Source: United Nations (*2*).

Group 1: countries in which a gradual decrease in the birth rate can be observed. Within this group some subcategories can be distinguished on the basis of the present level of fertility (initial and final values of the crude birth rate are shown alongside each country).

— Countries where fertility fell to a very low level:

Austria	19–12	Luxembourg	16–11
Belgium	17–12	Sweden	15–12
England	18–12	Switzerland	19–12
Federal Republic of Germany	18–10		

— Countries where fertility fell to a low level:

Denmark	17–13	Italy	18–13
Finland	18–14	Netherlands	21–13
France	18–14	Norway	17–13
Greece	18–16		

— Countries where fertility fell to a medium level:

Iceland	26–18	Spain	22–18
Malta	23–18	Yugoslavia	22–18
Portugal	24–18		

— Countries where fertility fell but remained at a high level:

Albania	38–30

Group 2: countries in which the birth rate did not change or changed very little.

Bulgaria	16–17	Ireland	22
Czechoslovakia	16–18		

Group 3: countries in which fertility increased continuously.

Hungary	14–16

Group 4: countries in which fertility first increased then decreased.

Romania	17–21–19

Group 5: countries in which fertility first decreased then increased.

Poland	20–17–19	USSR	22–17–18

Crude birth rates have remained high in Algeria, Morocco and Turkey. A certain decline can be discerned in all three countries between 1960–1964 and 1975–1979 but its extent was significant only in Turkey, where the rate fell by 15%. In the other two countries live-birth rates fell only by 6–9%. The rates for the five-year period 1975–1979 were estimated at 48 in Algeria, 45 in Morocco and 35 in Turkey per 1000 population.

The fluctuations in the crude birth rate in recent years can be seen from Table 2. In 1980, different trends were already evident in the European subregions. Compared with 1975, there was an increase of 2–3% in Western and Northern Europe. The crude birth rate did not change in the USSR but it fell by 18% in Southern Europe and by 4% in Eastern Europe. As a result, the relative levels in the regions changed slightly.

In this changing situation it is difficult to estimate fertility trends in the European countries even for the near future. If the medium variant population forecasts of the United Nations are considered (see Table 1), one sees that in the second half of the 1980s birth rates throughout Europe will be the same as in the 1970s. Thereafter, fertility is expected to decline by about 0.5 per 1000 over each five-year period, with the present level of 16 per 1000 falling to just over 14 per 1000 at the end of the century. This also means that, whereas between 1960 and 1980 live-birth rates decreased by one quarter in Europe, during the next 20 years (if one accepts this variant) they will fall by less than one tenth.

In Northern and Western Europe, which have the lowest rates at present, birth rates will presumably not change, while in Eastern Europe they are expected to fall by 18%, in Southern Europe by 14%, and in the USSR by 10%. As a result, the fertility levels of the different regions will become close to one another.

The projected rates are of course subject to error, with the uncertainties becoming greater and greater with time. On the basis of the low variant, there will be a gradual and then faster decrease so that by the end of the century the rate will have fallen by 19%. If, however, one accepts the high variant, fertility will rise by 4%. Examining the tendencies in Eastern and Southern Europe as well as in the USSR, a decline in live births is expected not only with the low variant but also with the high variant. At the same time in Northern and Western Europe the low variant projects a decrease and the high variant an increase. It must also be noted that for 1996–1999 the low variant of Western Europe shows the lowest crude birth rate (10 per 1000) and the high variant of the USSR the highest rate (17.5 per 1000).

The projections of live-birth rates for countries outside Europe are even more uncertain since even the present levels are estimates, not to mention that the future social, economic and cultural changes affecting the number of births are even less certain. However, the United Nations projections anticipate a very large decrease in live-birth rates in all three countries. According to the medium calculation, the live-birth rate will fall by 25% in Algeria, by 30% in Morocco and by 32% in Turkey. But even with such a decline in the two countries of North Africa, the number of live births

Table 2. Crude live-birth rates in Europe, 1975–1981

Region and country	1975	1976	1977	1978	1979	1980	1981
Eastern Europe							
Bulgaria	16.6	16.5	16.1	15.5	15.3	14.3	14.1
Czechoslovakia	19.6	19.2	18.7	18.4	17.8	16.2	15.5
German Democratic Republic	10.8	11.6	13.3	13.9	14.0	14.6	14.2
Hungary	18.4	17.5	16.7	15.7	15.0	13.9	13.3
Poland	18.9	19.5	19.1	19.0	19.5	19.5	18.9
Romania	19.7	19.5	19.5	19.1	18.5	18.0	17.0
Total	17.7	17.8	17.8	17.7	17.5	17.0	15.8
Northern Europe							
Denmark	14.2	12.9	12.2	12.2	11.6	11.2	10.4
Finland	13.9	14.1	13.9	13.5	13.3	13.1	13.2
Iceland	20.1	19.5	18.0	18.6	19.0	19.9	
Ireland	21.2	21.0	20.9	21.1	21.5	21.9	21.9
Norway	14.1	13.3	12.6	12.8	12.8	12.5	12.8
Sweden	12.6	12.0	11.6	11.2	11.6	11.7	11.3
United Kingdom	12.5	12.1	11.8	12.3	13.1	13.5	12.9
Total	13.1	12.7	12.3	12.6	13.2	13.4	13.0
Southern Europe							
Albania							
Greece	15.7	16.0	15.5	15.7	15.9	15.5	15.4
Italy	14.8	13.9	13.1	12.6	11.8	11.2	11.2
Malta	18.3	18.0	17.9	17.3	16.6	15.4	15.0
Portugal	19.1	19.3	18.6	17.1	16.3		
Spain	19.1	18.2	18.0	17.2	16.1	15.1	14.1
Yugoslavia	18.2	18.1	17.7	17.4	17.1	17.0	16.8
Total	17.2	16.6	16.1	15.5	14.7	14.1	13.5
Western Europe							
Austria	12.5	11.6	11.3	11.3	11.4	12.0	12.4
Belgium	12.2	12.3	12.4	12.4	12.6	12.7	12.6
France	14.1	13.6	14.0	13.8	14.1	14.8	14.9
Federal Republic of Germany	9.7	9.8	9.5	9.4	9.5	10.0	10.1
Luxembourg	11.2	11.0	11.4	11.4	11.2	11.5	
Netherlands	13.0	12.9	12.5	12.6	12.5	12.8	12.5
Switzerland	12.3	11.7	11.5	11.3	11.6	11.9	11.6
Total	12.0	11.8	11.8	11.7	11.8	12.4	12.3
Europe (except USSR)	15.0	14.7	14.5	14.3	14.2	14.1	13.6
USSR	18.2	18.5	18.1	18.3	18.3	18.3	18.7
Europe total	16.2	16.1	15.8	15.7	15.7	15.6	15.4

Source: United Nations (*3*).

per 1000 will still be very high (36 in Algeria, 32 in Morocco). Even the rate of 24 per 1000 expected for Turkey would still be about two thirds higher than the European average.

The Development of Total Fertility Rates

Actual changes in reproductive behaviour are better indicated by the total fertility rate (TFR) than by the trend in crude birth rates. The TFR indicates how many children a woman would give birth to in the course of her reproductive life, if the live-birth rates of the given period (year, five-year period) by age of mother did not change. At the same time it is also an indicator of generation replacement; a TFR of 2.1 corresponds roughly to replacement level, i.e. to a net reproduction rate of unity. In other words, a TFR of this value implies a sub-replacement level whereas a value of 2.2 or higher indicates prospective population growth.

The development of the TFR in Europe and its major regions can be seen in Table 3. It is clear that in Europe as a whole, a positive reproduction rate could still be observed until the middle of the 1970s; since then, however, the value has been below this level. Overall, the TFR declined by about one fifth between 1960–1964 and 1975–1979. In the next 20 years, however, according to the medium projections of the United Nations, it is not expected to change very much (a decline of only 4% is anticipated).

If one examines the development of this indicator by regions, it can be seen that Western and Northern Europe were the first regions to attain sub-replacement fertility, reaching this level by 1970–1974. According to the projections, this level will be attained in Southern Europe during the first half of the 1980s, and in Eastern Europe in the 1990s. The TFR in the USSR, however, is expected to exceed this level during the remainder of the century. In the last 20 years, the greatest decline was recorded in Western Europe: here the TFR declined by 40% during the period between 1960–1964 and 1975–1979. The decline was only marginally less in Northern Europe. In Southern Europe the TFR decreased by 17% on average, but declined by only 3% in Eastern Europe and by 6% in the USSR. During the next 20 years, however, a 6% increase in the TFR is projected for Western Europe, although little or no change is anticipated in Northern Europe and the USSR. Only in Southern and Eastern Europe will fertility continue to decrease (by 13% and 8% respectively).

The projection of the TFR is also uncertain, of course. However, there is a uniform expectation that in Northern and Western Europe in the 1990s the values of the low variant will not continue to decline — they are expected to stagnate at a very low level of 1.3–1.5 — and the values of the high variant (which is perhaps more probable) indicate a gradual increase. But even if this latter situation were to prove true, the values would still not be sufficient for replacement in these two regions by the end of the century. In Eastern Europe the low variant suggests a slow decline through to the first half of the 1990s, followed by stabilization of the rate at around 2.0; the high variant projects stability only at the end of the century. In Southern Europe the two values would develop in a similar way, but in addition the high value is

Table 3. Total fertility rates in the European Region, 1950–1999[a]

Region and country	1950–1954	1960–1964	1975–1979	1985–1989	1995–1999
Eastern Europe					
Bulgaria	2.5	2.2	2.3	2.2	2.1
Czechoslovakia	2.9	2.4	2.4	2.2	2.1
German Democratic Republic	2.4	2.5	1.8	1.7	1.8
Hungary	2.8	1.8	2.1	2.0	1.9
Poland	3.6	2.7	2.3	2.2	2.1
Romania	2.9	2.0	2.6	2.4	2.3
Total	3.0	2.3	2.3	2.2	2.1
Northern Europe					
Denmark	2.5	2.6	1.7	1.7	1.8
Finland	3.0	2.6	1.6	1.6	1.7
Iceland	3.7	3.9	2.3	1.9	1.9
Ireland	3.4	4.0	3.5	2.9	2.5
Norway	2.6	2.9	1.8	1.8	1.9
Sweden	2.2	2.3	1.7	1.5	1.7
United Kingdom	2.2	2.8	1.7	1.7	1.8
Total	2.3	2.8	1.8	1.7	1.8
Southern Europe					
Albania	5.6	5.7	4.2	3.1	2.4
Greece	2.3	2.2	2.3	2.3	2.3
Italy	2.3	2.6	1.9	1.8	1.7
Malta	4.1	3.1	2.0	2.0	2.0
Portugal	3.1	3.1	2.4	2.2	2.0
Spain	2.6	2.9	2.6	2.3	2.2
Yugoslavia	3.7	2.7	2.2	2.0	1.9
Total	2.7	2.7	2.3	2.0	2.0
Western Europe					
Austria	2.1	2.8	1.7	1.6	1.7
Belgium	2.4	2.7	1.7	1.7	1.8
France	2.7	2.9	1.9	1.8	1.8
Federal Republic of Germany	2.1	2.5	1.4	1.5	1.7
Luxembourg	2.0	2.4	1.6	1.5	1.6
Netherlands	3.1	3.1	1.6	1.6	1.8
Switzerland	2.3	2.5	1.5	1.5	1.6
Total	2.4	2.7	1.6	1.6	1.7
Europe (except USSR)	2.6	2.6	2.0	1.9	1.9
USSR	2.8	2.5	2.4	2.4	2.3
Europe total	2.7	2.6	2.1	2.1	2.0
Algeria			7.3	6.6	4.9
Morocco			6.9	5.7	4.1
Turkey			5.0	4.0	3.0

[a] Five-year averages. Projections based on United Nations medium variant as assessed in 1980.

Source: United Nations (*2*).

expected to fall slightly at the end of the century. In both regions the low values project a negative, and the high values a positive, reproduction level during the whole period. In the USSR the low fertility variants still imply a small positive reproduction level for the 1980s which is expected to stagnate in the 1990s; the high value, however, also promises stability here.

As is to be expected, the TFR in the three non-European countries of the Region is much higher than the level necessary for population replacement. In 1975–1979, an average of seven children per married woman was estimated for Algeria and Morocco and five for Turkey. In the first two countries mentioned, the family size corresponds to the level of natural fertility. According to the projections, however, TFRs are expected to decline substantially in all three countries by the end of the century. Even so, the average family size is expected to remain comparatively high with a TFR of about five in Algeria, four in Morocco and three in Turkey.

Age-specific Fertility Rates

To obtain a more precise insight into the changing pattern of fertility, it is necessary to examine trends in birth rates specific for the age of the mother. These are presented in Table 4 for 1960 and for the latest available year (in general 1977/1978).

For Europe as a whole, fertility in 1960 was highest at ages 25–29 years, but by the late 1970s the peak had shifted to 20–24 years. In recent years, in all age groups over 20 years, fertility has decreased, the extent of the decline increasing with age. Conversely, the fertility of 15–19-year-old females has risen by 7%.

In both periods under investigation (1960–1964 and 1975–1979) the age structure of fertility in Eastern Europe was markedly different from that in other European countries. The fertility of females under 25 years of age in Eastern Europe is much higher than the European average, and is also higher than that in other regions. Thus the fertility of females aged 15–19 years in Eastern Europe was nearly 90% higher than the European average in 1960 and nearly 70% higher in 1977–1978. For those aged 20–24 years the excess was 16% and 33%, respectively. In Western Europe the fertility of younger females is uniformly lower than the average. It is interesting to note that at the beginning of the 1960s Southern Europe was still characterized by a relatively high maternal age. However, by the late 1970s the relative fertility of women aged 15–24 years had increased significantly. A similar trend can be observed in the USSR. Quite the opposite occurred in the countries of Northern Europe. In 1960 the fertility of young females in these countries was relatively high; 18 years later, however, there was already a significant "deficit" compared with the overall European average. In Southern Europe and the USSR, the number of children born to females under 20 years of age rose substantially, while in Eastern Europe it remained largely unchanged. In Northern Europe it decreased by 40% and in Western Europe by one sixth. A similar trend can also be observed for the age group 20–24 years. These changes result from different fertility habits motivated primarily by the change in marriage habits.

Table 4. Live-birth rates in Europe, specific for age of mother, for different periods between 1959 and 1979

Region	Year	Age of mother (years)							
		15–49	15–19	20–24	25–29	30–34	35–39	40–44	45–49
Eastern Europe	1960	75.1	55.9	180.8	133.6	73.2	37.6	13.2	1.2
	1977/1978	70.4	53.9	184.1	123.3	64.2	22.2	5.5	0.4
Northern Europe	1960	73.1	46.6	159.5	168.7	103.7	51.2	16.4	1.2
	1977/1978	53.8	27.3	106.8	123.1	68.6	22.5	5.4	0.4
Southern Europe	1960	74.4	21.9	120.6	162.0	114.9	66.0	25.3	3.1
	1974/1978	66.3	31.5	133.8	145.4	90.5	42.7	14.1	1.4
Western Europe	1960	75.5	23.1	141.7	167.7	107.3	55.2	20.5	1.3
	1977/1978	48.7	19.3	100.0	116.9	63.8	20.2	5.0	0.4
Europe (except USSR)	1960	74.7	34.3	147.8	158.4	101.0	53.5	21.5	1.8
	1977/1978	59.5	32.0	131.0	127.4	72.2	27.4	7.7	0.7
USSR	1959	103.3	192.0		158.0	109.6	68.3	23.2	5.9
	1978/1979	69.9	39.4	174.6	125.6	72.1	31.9	11.7	1.6
Europe total	1959/1960	85.0	29.9	155.4	158.3	104.1	58.8	22.1	3.3
	1977/1979	63.1	34.6	146.3	126.8	72.2	29.0	9.1	1.0

Source: United Nations (*4*).

The fertility situation is quite different in the age group 25–34 years. In 1960 a distinct birth surplus was evident in Northern, Southern and Western Europe, whereas 18 years later this was characteristic only of Southern Europe. As a consequence of the early (age of mother) fertility in Eastern Europe, the number of children born to women in this age group is comparatively low.

The fertility of women over 35 years was highest in Southern Europe and the USSR at both dates. Here especially, the surplus fertility of 45–49-year-old women is significant: at both dates their fertility was three quarters higher than the average. Fertility in this age group has decreased in Northern and Western Europe but has remained unchanged in Eastern Europe. As a result, the greatest differences can be seen in the oldest age group: in 1960 the maximum was five times and in 1975–1977 eight times as high as the minimum.

As a consequence of these changes in age-specific fertility, there has been a shift in the distribution of births within the reproductive period. In 1960, some 65% of births were to mothers under 30 years of age. By the late 1970s this proportion had risen to 72%. Within this interval the proportion of births to 20–24-year-old women increased particularly rapidly, with the share of births to women under 20 years of age rising as well. The declining proportion of births to women over 30 years of age can be attributed mainly to a decline in the willingness of these women to give birth: over the period their share of births fell from 16% to 10%.

Although the differences between the regions have decreased somewhat, marked differences are still apparent. Eastern Europe is the region with the "youngest" fertility. At the same time the proportion of births at the younger ages is lowest in Southern Europe, although here a significant rise can be observed. The share of births to mothers under 30 years of age also increased in the other regions. In Eastern Europe the proportion of births to mothers under 20 years of age was highest at both dates and is still high in Northern Europe.

Conversely, the proportion of births to mothers over 30 years of age declined in all regions; the number of births to those over 30 years of age is still the lowest in Eastern Europe. The highest proportion of births in this age group occurred in Southern Europe at both dates, though here, too, it decreased quite substantially. The difference among the regions is greatest in the proportion of births to women over 35 years of age; this is lowest in Eastern and Northern Europe, and highest in Southern Europe and in the USSR. Interestingly, the proportion has increased in three countries — Belgium, France and Luxembourg — over the last 15 years but decreased by over one third in two neighbouring countries, the Netherlands and Switzerland.

The development of fertility trends presented here on the basis of total fertility rates at different dates yields practically the same results as if a finer method of analysis is used. Thus if the total fertility of the individual female cohorts who accounted for the majority of births in the previous decades is studied, a similar tendency is found. If in some selected countries a comparison of completed fertility of birth cohorts is made, one finds that the fertility of the 1920 cohort was lower than that of the 1930 and 1940 cohorts in some countries, but that the fertility of the 1950 cohort — which exerts the greatest impact on current fertility — is lowest everywhere in Europe. In other countries, especially in Italy and the Netherlands, a gradual decrease can be observed (see Table 5).

Table 5. Completed fertility of female birth cohorts in six European countries — average total numbers of children

Country	Female birth cohort			
	1920	1930	1940	1950
England & Wales	2.00	2.33	2.35	2.12
France	2.50	2.64	2.41	2.06
Federal Republic of Germany	1.90	2.14	1.98	1.67
Italy	2.44	2.24	2.11	1.88
Netherlands	3.06	2.67	2.24	1.84
Sweden	2.14	2.10	2.07	1.98

Source: Calot, G. & Blayo, C., unpublished data, 1981.

Differential Fertility

In addition to the general level of fertility, the investigation of differences in fertility by socioeconomic status and cultural level, as well as of trends in these differences, is of considerable importance for understanding developments in fertility. This analysis is difficult to make on a regional level because of lack of comparable data, although some general conclusions can be drawn.

From the findings of the fertility surveys around 1970 shown in Tables 6 and 7, in all countries for which data are available there are large differences in the total expected number of children, both by socio-occupational status of the husband and by the educational level of the wife. But the size of the differences arouses further reflection: although the total fertility of married women whose husbands belong to the non-agricultural, non-manual socio-occupational group is the lowest everywhere, it differs considerably from the total fertility of those belonging to the agricultural manual group, who have the highest fertility. Similarly there are rather large differences in fertility between mothers with the highest and lowest educational levels.

Table 6. Average total numbers of children expected, by socio-occupational status of the husband

Country	Socio-occupational status of husband						
	Non-agricultural, non-manual		Non-agricultural, manual			Agricultural	
	High level	Other	Skilled	Semi-skilled	Un-skilled	Farmer	Farm worker
Belgium	2.7	2.2	2.4	2.5	2.5	3.0	
Czechoslovakia	2.2		2.5			2.9	
Denmark	2.5	2.4	2.4	2.5		2.9	2.9
England & Wales	2.1	2.0	2.2	2.4	2.6	2.8	2.7
Finland	2.4		2.5			2.8	
France	2.7	2.4	2.5	2.7	3.0	2.8	3.5
Hungary	1.9	1.8	2.1	2.5		2.1	2.5
Poland	2.2		2.8			3.6	3.5
Turkey	4.1	5.0	4.7	5.9	5.5	6.6	6.3
Yugoslavia	2.3		2.7			3.0	

Source: United Nations (*5*).

Table 7. Average total numbers of children expected, by educational level of the wife

Country	Educational level of wife				
	Less than elementary	Elementary	Lower secondary	Higher secondary	Post-secondary
Belgium	3.3	2.5	2.5	2.4	2.8
Czechoslovakia	2.6		2.1		2.1
Denmark	2.6		2.4	2.5	2.7
England & Wales		2.2		2.1	2.1
Finland	2.6		2.2		2.5
France	4.1	2.7	2.3	2.4	2.4
Hungary	3.6	2.5	2.2	1.9	1.9
Poland	3.1	3.3	2.8	2.3	2.0
Turkey	5.8	3.8	3.3	2.4	
Yugoslavia	3.4	2.5	2.3	1.9	1.9

Source: United Nations (*5*).

There is evidence to suggest that cultural changes are responsible for the general decline in fertility level. This is well established by the fertility of individual female cohorts in Hungary. From these data it is clear that if the educational level had not changed, i.e. if the standardized fertility indicators are taken as a basis for comparison, the level of completed fertility would scarcely have changed. In other words, the change in fertility cannot be attributed in the majority of cases to the fall in the actual fertility level within social strata but to the sociocultural restratification itself (see Table 8). As this process is likely to continue, if the fertility "deficit" of females with a higher education does not cease, a similar trend can be anticipated for the future.

Table 8. Average number of children by educational level of married women in Hungary, 1960–1980

Year	Educational level					Total
	Elementary (years)			Secondary	Post-secondary	
	≦5	6–7	8			
Average number of children born						
1960	3.26	2.39	1.41	1.29	1.28	2.32
1970	3.11	2.36	1.52	1.18	1.23	2.05[a]
1980	2.99	2.24	1.71	1.38	1.36	1.88[a]
Percentage of women						
1960	24	49	22	4	1	100
1970	16	38	34	10	2	100
1980	9	25	43	18	5	100

[a] When standardized by the educational level of 1960, the value for 1970 is 2.30 and for 1980 is 2.26.

Source: Klinger, A., unpublished data, 1981.

The data for England & Wales clearly show the changes in fertility that have occurred in the different socioeconomic groups in recent years. As can be seen from Table 9, the decline in fertility varied for the different strata and this decrease was greatest for those groups having a higher fertility. This is well reflected in reduction in fertility of those groups with higher parity.

Table 9. Estimated legitimate live births by social class of husband and number of previous live-born children, 1975 (England & Wales)

Social class of husband	Total	Number of previous live-born children			
		0	1	2	3 or more
Number in 1975 (thousands)					
All classes	549	228	204	73	44
Total non-manual	199	88	78	23	10
I and II	142	61	56	17	8
III N	57	27	22	6	2
Total manual	350	140	126	50	34
III M	214	85	80	30	19
IV and V	136	55	46	20	15
1975 Index (1970 = 100)					
All classes	76	83	86	62	49
Total non-manual	89	94	98	65	58
I and II	96	104	107	67	64
III N	75	78	81	60	46
Total manual	70	76	78	60	46
III M	71	77	81	60	45
IV and V	67	74	73	59	48

Source: Fox, J., unpublished data, 1981.

Parity

The age of the mother is closely related to the birth order of live births. This distribution is presented in Table 10 which shows quite clearly that, in parallel with the reduction in fertility in Europe, the proportion of first-born children and then that of second-born children increased. Conversely the proportion of higher order, and especially of the fifth and subsequent births, decreased. Between 1963 and 1978/1979 in Europe, the proportion of infants of the fourth and higher birth orders fell by more than two thirds and that of the third birth order declined by more than one fifth. By 1978/1979 some 45% of births were first births, compared with only 37% in 1963.

Studying the distribution by birth order in the individual regions, one can see that in 1978 the proportion of first-born children was highest in Western Europe and in the USSR (46% of all births). This was some 10% more than that prevailing 15 years earlier. In the three other regions the proportion of first-born infants is 42–44%. The proportion of second births is more balanced and has grown by almost the same amount. It is interesting to note that in 1963 children of birth order three were relatively more common in Northern and Western Europe (16–17% of births), whereas in the three other regions the proportion was 14%. Currently, the proportion

Table 10. Percentage distribution of live births by birth order and legitimacy in Europe in different periods between 1963 and 1979

Region	Year	Birth order					Total	Per cent illegitimate
		1st	2nd	3rd	4th	5th+		
Eastern Europe	1963	39	30	14	7	10	100	5.7[a]
	1978/1979	44	35	12	5	4	100	10.1[a]
Northern Europe	1963	36	31	17	8	8	100	7.1
	1976/1979	42	38	13	4	3	100	14.2
Southern Europe	1963	37	28	14	8	13	100[b]	3.5
	1976/1979	42	33	13	6	6	100	4.1
Western Europe	1963	37	28	16	8	11	100	5.2
	1978/1979	46	35	12	4	3	100	8.0
Europe (except USSR)	1963	37	29	15	8	11	100[b]	5.2[a]
	1978/1979	44	35	12	5	4	100	8.4[a]
USSR	1963	36	28	14	8	14	100	
	1978	46	30	10	5	9	100	
Europe total	1963	37	29	14	8	12	100[b]	
	1978/1979	45	33	11	5	6	100	

[a] Excluding Romania.

[b] Excluding Malta and Spain.

Source: United Nations (*6*).

of third-order births is lowest in the USSR (10%) and in the other four regions there is scarcely any difference (12–13%). Fourth and higher order births were proportionately highest in the USSR in both years (22% and 14%, respectively) and in 1978/1979 were least common in Northern and Western Europe (7% of all births).

Legitimacy

Table 10 also shows the distribution of live births by legitimacy in Europe, except for the USSR where such data are not available. The proportion of "illegitimate" births has increased considerably in Europe. This category includes not only those children who were born "out-of-wedlock" in the traditional sense of the word but also those who were born to a couple cohabiting but not formally married. Between 1963 and 1978/1979 the proportion of such births grew from 5.2% to 8.4%, i.e. by more than 60%. The proportion is highest in Northern Europe where 14% of babies are born illegitimate, and in ten years the proportion has doubled. In Eastern Europe the proportion has increased by three quarters and in Western Europe by half. Only in Southern Europe — where illegitimacy was always comparatively rare — can a slight decrease be discerned.

The proportion of illegitimate births and the increase in this proportion have developed in different ways within the individual regions. There are countries for which this phenomenon is especially characteristic, and it may therefore cause some social and perhaps also health problems. Table 11 shows the European countries with the highest proportions of illegitimate births in 1978/1979, and compares these rates with those in 1963.

Table 11. European countries with the highest proportions of illegitimate births in 1978/1979 and the corresponding rates for 1963

Country	Illegitimate births as a percentage of all births in:	
	1978/1979	1963
Sweden	38	13
Iceland	37	25
Denmark	31	9
German Democratic Republic	20	9
Austria	15	12
Norway	13	4
Finland	12	4
France	10	6
England	10	7
Bulgaria	10	8

There are countries, however, where this situation is relatively unknown. According to recent data, only 1% of newborn babies are illegitimate in Greece and Malta, and only about 2–3% in Belgium, Italy, the Netherlands and Spain.

Desired Family Size

Table 12 summarizes information about desired family size in the European countries for which survey data are available. From studies carried out between 1975 and 1977, the average desired number of children varied between 1.9 (Bulgaria) and 2.8 (Spain). Comparatively low desired family size was also reported for Hungary (2.0), Great Britain (2.3) and Flanders (2.3). The average desired number of children in the other countries listed was between 2.4 and 2.7. This clearly shows that the desired family size of married women is much higher than the number of children realized, measured either by total fertility rates or on the basis of the completed fertility rate as calculated from the population censuses. In some countries for which fertility data from the 1970 round of population censuses are available, completed fertility has developed as shown in Table 13.

Table 12. Distribution of married women of reproductive age, by number of children desired

Country	Year of survey	Percentage distribution by desired complete family size						Average number desired
		0	1	2	3	4	5+	
Belgium (Flanders)	1966	6	21	34	20	11	8	2.39
	1975	4	19	43	21	9	4	2.25
Bulgaria	1976	11	21	51	11	3	3	1.86
Czechoslovakia	1970	1	9	58	23	5	4	2.37
	1977	3	9	50	26	8	3	2.46
Denmark	1970	3	8	43	31	11	4	2.55
England & Wales	1967	8	19	41	18	9	5	2.21
Finland	1971	3	10	47	23	10	7	2.55
	1977	3	10	45	28	10	4	2.46
France	1971	3	14	40	25	11	7	2.55
	1976	3	13	41	28	8	7	2.54
Great Britain	1976	4	12	50	21	9	4	2.32
Hungary	1965	3	20	50	17	6	4	2.19
	1977	2	15	64	15	3	1	2.08
Italy	1979	1	13	49	25	7	5	2.40
Norway	1977	4	7	45	30	11	3	2.49
Poland	1972	2	9	40	27	12	10	2.80
	1977	1	10	50	26	8	5	2.50
Romania	1978	3	9	59	18	11		2.22
Spain	1977	1	6	43	28	12	9	2.80
Yugoslavia	1970	...	...	...	...	...	...	2.82
	1976	...	...	...	...	...	...	2.73

Source: Leridon, H. (*7*); World Fertility Survey (*8*); Demographic Research Centre (*9*).

Table 13. Number of children born alive per 100 married women aged 45–49 years

Country	Number of children
German Democratic Republic	186
Federal Republic of Germany	193
Luxembourg	204
Hungary	214
Belgium	219
Czechoslovakia	235
Bulgaria	250
Romania	273
Yugoslavia	285
Portugal	291
Spain	292
Poland	312
Ireland	429

The differences between the countries can be ascribed mainly to the various desires relating to family size. In general, married women everywhere desire most frequently a two-child family. Nonetheless, some important variations still exist between countries. In Hungary, 65% of married women desire two children, and in Czechoslovakia also the proportion is quite high (58%) according to the 1970 survey. Around half the number of married women interviewed in Great Britain and Poland want two children, while in Denmark, France and Spain the figure is only 43%.

There are also interesting intercountry differences in the desire to have three children. The lowest proportion of married women wanting this number is found in Hungary (13%), and the maximum in Denmark and Spain (31–32%); the figures for France and Poland are also high. Given the actual fertility, some of these desired family size figures seem unrealistic. This also applies to the idea of a "large family" consisting of four or more children; this will probably not be realized for the 15% of married women in Denmark and France or the 20% in Spain who reported such a desired family size. In Hungary, however, the proportion of those desiring four or more children was only 3%.

The differences are similar in the desire for only one child. This was most frequently reported among Belgian women (21% in 1966), somewhat less frequently in Hungary (17%) and still rather frequently in France and Great Britain (13%). In Spain the proportion was only 4%. This desired family size was also unrealistically low in the other countries of the region, where only about 7–9% of women wanted one child. In actual fact, the share of one-child families has been increasing everywhere as has the proportion of childless families, which are rarely planned but which for health (infertility) and other reasons are rather frequent.

Family Planning

Contraceptive behaviour

The survey data also yield information on the spread of birth control and on the method used. The figures are shown in Table 14. Here attention should be drawn first of all to the differences in the proportion of users. According to the data available from the recent surveys, in Europe the ratio of non-users varies between 50% (Spain) and 12–13% (Czechoslovakia and Flanders). Non-use is also low in France (18%) and comparatively high in Yugoslavia (39%); use in the other countries varies between 22% and 30%. Among non-users the proportion of pregnant females varies between 4% and 9%, and of women seeking pregnancy from 4% to 7%. A significant proportion of non-users (2–7%) are infertile. The differences in the proportion of females who consciously do not use any form of contraception are much greater. According to the data available, around 10% of married women of reproductive age in Denmark, Great Britain, Hungary and the Netherlands fall into this category, rising to over one quarter in Yugoslavia and to nearly half of all married women in Spain.

Among users, those using a reversible method form the majority in all countries. There are very great differences in the use of various methods. By the middle of the 1970s, modern contraceptive methods prevailed in many countries and of these the Pill was the most frequently used. Among married women of reproductive age, the proportion using oral contraception was 46% in the Netherlands,[a] 36% in Hungary, 32% in Flanders, 27% in France and 24% in Great Britain. However, this method was used less often in Czechoslovakia and Spain (11%) and was even less popular in Yugoslavia (4%). In these last three countries traditional methods are generally used because effective modern methods are less easily available. The proportion of women using such methods, of the total number of females of reproductive age, was 56% in Czechoslovakia, 45% in Yugoslavia and 31% in Spain. But it was also high in Flanders and France (31–36%). Of these methods withdrawal is especially common, although its efficacy in family planning is very low; 34–35% of couples still use this contraceptive method in Czechoslovakia and Yugoslavia, 30% in Flanders, France and Spain, and 17% in Hungary. However, only 2% in the Netherlands use withdrawal and 4–6% in Denmark, Great Britain and Norway.

From the data in Table 14 it can be seen that in some European countries sterilization as a means of family planning is becoming more common. Whilst it is not always clear whether sterilization — either of the wife or of the husband — is carried out for contraceptive reasons, the incidence of sterilization has in some countries increased considerably compared with the mid-1960s, and its role in family planning and its impact on fertility will increase even more in the future. According to the data available, the frequency of sterilization is greatest in Denmark and Great Britain, where at

[a] Only for women married during the period 1963–1973.

Table 14. Percentage of contraceptive use among married women of reproductive age

Country	Year of survey	Currently using reversible method					Sterilized	Non-users
		Pill	IUD	Condom	Other	Total		
Belgium (Flanders)	1966	5	0	4	67	76	3	21
	1975/1976	32	4	9	36	81	6	13
Bulgaria	1976	2	2	2	70	76	2	24
Czechoslovakia	1970	3	9	12	42	66	—	34
	1977	11	17	13	56	85	3	12
Denmark	1970	25	3	20	19	67	0	33
	1975	19	8	22	9	58	19	23
England & Wales	1967	13	1	28	27	69	4	27
Finland	1971	20	3	31	23	77	—	23
	1977	11	28	32	5	76	4	20
Great Britain	1976	24	6	18	10	58	19	23
France	1971	11	1	7	45	64	5	31
	1978	27	10	6	31	74	8	18
Hungary	1965/1966	0	0	10	54	64	0	36
	1977	36	10	4	23	73	0	27
Italy	1979	13	2	13	49	77	1	22
Netherlands	1969	27	1	13	18	59	0	41
	1975	46	4	10	6	66	4	30
Norway	1977	16	28	15	12	71	7	22
Poland	1972	2	1	10	47	60	...	40
	1977	8	1	14	52	75	...	25
Romania	1978	1	...	3	54	58	...	42
Spain	1977	11	0	5	31	47	3	50
Yugoslavia	1970	5	1	3	50	59	...	41
	1976	4	2	2	45	53	8	39

Source: Leridon, H. (*7*); World Fertility Survey (*8*); Demographic Research Centre (*9*).

least one of the spouses has been sterilized in nearly one fifth of couples. The extent of sterilization is also fairly high (6–8%) in Belgium, France, Norway and Yugoslavia.

Induced abortion

In addition to contraceptive practice, the level and pattern of fertility is also influenced by the incidence of induced abortion. The legalization of abortion is becoming increasingly common in European countries, having been introduced in recent years in several countries of Western and Southern Europe. In the majority of countries of Eastern Europe and in the USSR, measures to legalize abortion were taken in the mid-1950s, and in the Scandinavian countries even earlier. In the mid-1960s and the early 1970s these countries — except the German Democratic Republic where abortion was legalized only during that period — restricted induced abortion to a certain extent. In most of the Scandinavian countries, however, the regulations were later relaxed again.

These changing legal regulations exerted a considerable influence on the incidence of induced abortions. According to Table 15, both the abortion rates and the abortion ratios generally decreased in the countries of Eastern Europe but increased in Northern Europe during the 1970s. The data, of course, refer only to legal abortions. It is difficult to estimate the total number of abortions and therefore the impact of legislation on that total.

Table 15. Legal induced abortion rates and ratios in Europe, 1960–1979[a]

Country	Abortion rate per 1000 women aged 15–44 years				Abortion ratio per 100 live births			
	1960–1964	1965–1969	1970–1974	1975–1979	1960–1964	1965–1969	1970–1974	1975–1979
Eastern Europe								
Bulgaria	41.5	53.6	66.5	66.1[b]	57.0	76.7	90.2	88.2[b]
Czechoslovakia	29.2	30.6	29.0	27.9	36.6	42.6	34.8	32.2
German Democratic Republic	—	—	31.4[b]	23.7[b]	—	—	59.0[b]	40.3[b]
Hungary	78.3	85.1	72.0	39.1	127.1	130.1	104.7	51.7
Poland[c]	...	21.9	18.4	17.9[b]	...	29.5	23.7	21.5[b]
Romania[d]	222.1	124.5	74.4	83.1	314.7	169.9	81.2	92.4
Northern Europe								
Denmark	4.3	6.2	14.8	24.2	5.1	7.9	20.6	40.6
Finland	5.6[b]	6.1[b]	19.5	17.2	7.1[b]	14.9[b]	34.2	29.0[b]
Iceland	...	...	4.3[b]	8.6[b]	...	...	4.4[b]	10.1[b]
Norway	...	8.1[b]	15.9	18.9	...	8.8[b]	19.3	28.7
Sweden	2.1[b]	5.2[b]	14.6	20.0	2.9[b]	7.1[b]	21.1	34.2
United Kingdom: England & Wales	—	4.4[b]	10.6	11.1	—	5.2	14.5	18.0
Southern Europe								
Italy	—	—	—	15.8[b]	—	—	—	28.8[b]
Yugoslavia	34.2[b]	42.7	47.8[b]	...	37.8[b]	51.3	69.9[b]	...
Western Europe								
France	—	—	—	13.2[b]	—	—	—	19.9[b]
Federal Republic of Germany	—	—	—	5.3[b]	—	—	—	12.0[b]
Netherlands[e]	—	—	6.8[b]	5.2	—	—	10.0[b]	8.9

[a] Five-year averages.

[b] The data are for part of the quinquennium only.

[c] Abortions carried out in hospitals and clinics.

[d] Legal abortions and spontaneous abortions requiring hospital treatment.

[e] Residents only.

Source: Tietze, C. (*10*).

With the greater application of family planning methods some risk to health may arise, though the risk will be less than that associated with pregnancy. However, in recent years, a number of studies have demonstrated that induced abortion — especially repeated abortions and those carried out at a late stage of pregnancy, or if the abortion is not performed by a specialist and/or not performed in hospital — has significant side effects. These often consist of minor infections which, though quite prevalent, are generally curable. In general, however, a previous induced abortion greatly increases the incidence of premature birth during a later pregnancy. Similarly, secondary sterility is more frequent following an induced abortion. It is therefore desirable that the number of induced abortions be kept to a minimum, especially prior to the first birth. Legislation to this effect has been enacted in several countries.

Health risks have also been identified among women who use oral contraceptives for a long period. This has been found to lead to disease later in life. Thus, among women over 35 years of age who take hormonal contraceptives, the incidence of certain diseases of the circulatory system is higher, the risk increasing if the woman also has high blood pressure and/or smokes cigarettes. At younger ages, the use of such contraceptives might lead to hormonal irregularities. It is therefore imperative that the choice of contraceptive method be made in relation to the woman's age, parity and lifestyle, and health education must be broadened to promote alternative contraceptive methods.

Conclusions for Health Policy

Fertility trends in Europe over the next few decades are likely to have the following social and health implications which should be taken into consideration in the development of social and health policy.

- Low fertility will continue, which will further increase the number of families with few children. The number of large families will continue to be low but their socioeconomic circumstances may worsen. Social and health policy must therefore treat these families as a separate and urgent case.

- Parallel with the decline in fertility the number of older mothers has fallen. From the health viewpoint this is a positive development because babies born to older mothers are more at risk. At the same time the proportion of young mothers — those under 20 years of age — has increased, most of them bearing children outside marriage. Risks to the health of both mother and child are also greater at these ages. More attention must therefore be paid to the case of women in this age group, especially to prevent unplanned pregnancies and to improve the survival chances of the infant.

- The modernization of family planning methods and the spread of the most efficacious and less dangerous methods has contributed to the decrease in the number of unplanned pregnancies. The use of more dangerous methods such as abortion should be discouraged, both for health reasons and to reduce subsequent infertility.

References

1. **Klinger, A.** On the fertility of the developed countries. *Demografia,* **23**: 337 (1980).
2. *Selected demographic indicators by country, 1950–2000.* New York, United Nations, 1980; *World population prospects as assessed in 1980.* New York, United Nations, 1981.
3. *Monthly bulletin of statistics.* New York, United Nations, September 1981.
4. *Demographic yearbook. Special issue: historical supplement.* New York, United Nations, 1979; *Demographic yearbook, 1979.* New York, United Nations, 1981.
5. *Fertility and family planning in Europe around 1970.* New York, United Nations, 1976.
6. *Demographic yearbook, 1969 and 1975.* New York, United Nations, 1970, 1976.
7. **Leridon, H.** Fertility and contraception in 12 developed countries. *International family planning perspectives,* **7**(2): 70–78 (1981).
8. *The Czechoslovak fertility survey, 1977.* London, World Fertility Survey, 1978.
9. *Fertility and family planning in Yugoslavia.* Belgrade, Demographic Research Centre, 1980.
10. **Tietze, C.** *Induced abortion, a world review.* New York, Population Council, 1981.

4

Trends and perspectives in mortality

E. Lynge

The European Region is especially suitable for mortality studies because all countries have well established civil registration systems and regularly publish mortality statistics. Most European countries are demographically in the post-transitional stage, and the overall level of mortality is low compared with other parts of the world. Important knowledge about determinants of human health has been gained through studies of the decline in mortality in Europe in the nineteenth and the first half of the twentieth centuries. Perhaps the most outstanding feature of this process is the elimination of tuberculosis as a cause of death due to better dietary and sanitary conditions (*1*).

Although the present changes in mortality in Europe are less dramatic, important clues about determinants of health can still be generated through studies of recent trends and differentials in mortality. Thus, despite the low mortality levels — and the generally still declining trends in mortality — adverse trends do occur and constant monitoring of mortality rates is necessary to quickly identify such changes. It is also important to remember that low mortality is not equivalent to complete survival; some babies still die, and a happy retirement is still experienced by only a proportion of the population. Studies of differentials in mortality serve to identify the risk factors that underlie these premature deaths.

The main purpose of mortality studies in Europe today is thus to prevent any deterioration in survival chances and to help identify and eliminate risk factors. However, there are several steps between the purely demographic description and suggestions for specific preventive measures. The description may reveal patterns of mortality, the patterns may lead to the generation of hypotheses about risk factors, and the suspicions may be followed up in hypothesis-testing studies. But even factors confirmed to be dangerous to human health may not necessarily be eliminated, e.g. a carcinogenic chemical may still be used for economic reasons. Therefore, whereas it is the job of scientists to carry out the analyses of mortality, it is the task of society to take the political decisions on interventions.

Inasmuch as the decline in mortality in Europe first began to cease in some countries in the late 1950s, a thorough analysis of mortality trends in all European countries over the period 1950–1980 by sex, age and specific causes of death would be highly valuable. Such an extensive investigation has been attempted elsewhere (*2*) and is beyond the scope of this chapter. Rather, the focus here is on selected patterns of mortality that should be further investigated to improve understanding of the determinants of health.

Mortality Differentials in Europe

Regional differences

Life expectancy at birth for the sexes during the years 1977 and 1978 is given in Table 1 for all European countries[a] with the exception of Albania and the European part of the USSR. The life expectancy at birth for males in 1977/1978 was over 70 years in 9 of the 28 countries. Furthermore, there is no simple geographical gradient in mortality. Although life expectancy is almost equal in Norway (72.4 years), Sweden (72.5 years) and Greece (72.9 years) the age-specific death rates differ markedly; infant mortality is lower in Scandinavia than in Greece, but from age 40 onwards the opposite is true. The high life expectancy for men in Greece has led to questions about the validity of the statistics. According to the Greek report there would appear to be some under-registration of infant deaths, especially in the rural areas. However, this does not explain why life expectancy for females in Greece is closer to the life expectancy in the surrounding countries than is the case for men.

The life expectancy for women exceeds 70 years in all countries, and is over 78 years in five countries. Iceland, the Netherlands, Norway, Sweden and Switzerland all have a life expectancy for men exceeding 70 years and a life expectancy for women exceeding 78 years.

The lowest life expectancy at birth for males is found in Portugal (65.1 years in 1975). Portugal is also among the countries with the lowest life expectancy for women. In Table 2 age-standardized death rates for main causes are compared for Portugal and Sweden, the latter representing countries with low mortality. However, it is difficult to conclude which diseases contribute to the excess mortality in Portugal, because deaths due to senility and ill-defined causes account for nearly half the excess. Only respiratory diseases can be identified as a main contributor.

The difference in mortality between Finland and Sweden is remarkable. In 1961–1965 the difference in life expectancy for men was 6.2 years (*5*). The

---

[a] The figures in Table 1 are taken primarily from the *World health statistics annual* (*3*) but some have been taken from the United Nations *Demographic yearbook* (*4*). The two sources are not totally comparable; for example the life expectancy for Hungarian men in 1978 is 66.1 years in the first and 66.6 years in the second, which is a variation of the same order as the real differences we are interested in detecting.

Table 1. Expectation of life at birth and at 45 years of age, by sex

Country	Year	Expectation of life at birth		Expectation of life at 45 years of age	
		Males	Females	Males	Females
Austria	1978	68.4	75.7	27.7	33.2
Belgium	1976	68.9	75.5	27.8	33.1
Bulgaria	1977	68.2	73.5	28.0	31.7
Czechoslovakia	1975	67.2	73.6	26.5	31.9
	1977*	66.99	74.12	—	—
Denmark	1978	71.7	77.7	29.5	34.7
Finland	1975	67.4	76.3	26.4	33.4
	1978*	68.49	77.12	26.77	33.81
France	1976	69.9	77.9	28.6	35.3
	1977*	69.73	77.85	28.60	35.25
German Democratic Republic	1976	68.9	74.5	27.7	31.9
Germany, Federal Republic of	1978	69.2	76.0	28.1	33.6
Greece	1978	72.9	77.6	31.6	35.2
Hungary	1978	66.1	72.8	26.0	31.0
	1978*	66.62	73.26	26.55	31.51
Iceland	1978	73.8	80.0	32.7	37.0
Ireland	1975	69.0	74.3	27.7	31.8
Italy	1975	69.8	76.1	28.6	33.8
Luxembourg	1978	68.3	75.8	27.0	32.8
Malta	1977	68.8	72.6	26.6	30.4
Netherlands	1978	72.0	78.7	29.7	35.7
Norway	1978	72.4	78.8	30.2	35.6
Poland	1978	66.5	74.9	26.8	33.0
Portugal	1975	65.1	72.6	27.3	32.4
Romania	1978	67.3	72.4	28.1	31.7
Spain	1976	70.8	76.7	29.5	34.2
Sweden	1978	72.5	79.0	30.4	35.8
Switzerland	1978	72.0	78.9	30.2	35.8
United Kingdom:					
England & Wales	1977	70.2	76.3	28.2	33.6
Northern Ireland	1977	67.5	74.1	26.5	31.9
Scotland	1978	68.2	74.4	26.5	31.8
Yugoslavia	1977	67.8	73.0	28.4	32.4

Source: World Health Organization (*3*); entries marked* are taken from the United Nations (*4*).

Table 2. Age-standardized mortality rates (per 10 000) by cause of death in Sweden and Portugal, 1975

Cause of death	Men			Women		
	Sweden (S)	Portugal (P)	Difference (P–S)	Sweden (S)	Portugal (P)	Difference (P–S)
Infectious diseases	0.7	3.4	2.7	0.4	1.8	1.4
Malignant neoplasms	17.8	15.0	- 2.8	13.2	9.9	- 3.3
Circulatory diseases	41.9	45.4	3.5	35.5	33.4	- 2.1
Respiratory diseases	4.4	13.0	8.6	2.4	7.3	4.9
Digestive diseases	3.8	8.0	4.2	2.1	3.5	1.4
Genitourinary diseases	1.5	2.1	0.6	0.8	1.0	0.2
Senility; ill-defined symptoms	0.4	16.7	16.3	0.3	14.7	14.4
Accidents	8.5	11.5	3.0	3.8	3.0	- 0.8
Other	5.2	6.8	1.6	4.4	5.2	0.8
Total	84.3	121.9	37.6	62.9	79.9	17.0

Source: Caselli, G. & Egidi, V. (*2*).

most recent figures from 1978 show a difference of 4.0 years (Table 1). The difference in life expectancy for women is also decreasing and was 1.9 years in 1978. In 1978 Finnish males had an excess mortality compared with Swedish males from age 5 and onwards, whereas the excess for Finnish women in comparison with their Swedish counterparts was restricted to ages 55 and over.

Table 3 shows the age-standardized death rates from the main causes of death for men and women in Finland and Sweden (*5*). It is apparent that all main causes contribute to the excess in mortality among Finnish men. Considerable differences in mortality within Finland are also evident. Indeed, the difference in life expectancy between the western coastal area with low mortality and the eastern Karelia area with high mortality is of the same order as that between Finland and Sweden (Central Statistical Office of Finland, unpublished data, 1981).

Table 3. Age-standardized mortality rates (per 100 000) by main causes of death in Finland and Sweden, 1971–1975

Cause of death	Men		Women	
	Finland	Sweden	Finland	Sweden
Circulatory diseases	501	338	276	202
Malignant neoplasms	185	144	99	112
Other diseases	184	130	114	87
Violent death	135	83	36	33
Total	1 005	696	526	434

Source: Nordic Statistical Secretariat (*5*).

Sex differences

Women have a higher life expectancy than men in all European countries — on average about 6.5 years more. The difference is less than 6 years in Malta (3.8 years), Greece (4.7 years), Romania (5.1 years), Yugoslavia (5.2 years), Bulgaria and Ireland (5.3 years) and the German Democratic Republic (5.6 years). It is over 7 years in Finland (8.6 years), Poland (8.4 years), France (8.1 years), Luxembourg and Portugal (7.5 years), Austria (7.3 years) and Czechoslovakia (7.1 years). There seems to be a concentration of small sex differences in the south-eastern part of Europe.

In Table 4 age-standardized death rates by main causes of death are compared for men and women in France and Greece (*2*). The age-standardized death rates for women in France are considerably below the

Table 4. Age-standardized mortality rates (per 10 000) by cause of death in France and Greece, 1975

Cause of death	France (1974–1976)			Greece (1975–1976)		
	Men	Women	Female mortality as a percentage of male mortality	Men	Women	Female mortality as a percentage of male mortality
Infectious diseases	1.7	0.9	53	1.6	1.0	63
Malignant neoplasms	23.3	12.2	52	16.2	9.2	57
Circulatory diseases	32.6	20.3	62	26.5	22.1	83
Respiratory diseases	6.9	3.4	49	7.4	5.2	70
Digestive diseases	7.3	3.4	47	3.6	1.9	53
Genitourinary diseases	1.7	0.7	41	2.2	1.3	59
Senility; ill-defined symptoms	6.5	4.6	71	6.5	6.5	100
Accidents	11.3	4.9	43	5.7	2.6	46
Other	7.2	5.6	78	8.1	7.5	93
Total	98.4	55.9		77.8	57.4	

Source: Caselli, G. & Egidi, V. (*2*).

rates for men for all main causes of death (except for senility and ill-defined symptoms and for other causes of death). It is therefore a broad spectrum of diseases that contribute to the excess mortality for men in France. Table 4 also shows that the comparatively small differential in life expectancy between men and women in Greece is the result of small differences in mortality for all causes of death. Yet even in Greece, the female death rates for cancer, digestive diseases and accidents are only half the male death rates.

The widening sex difference in life expectancy is one of the striking features of mortality in Europe. This trend has had a considerable influence on the sex composition of the elderly.

Socioeconomic differences

The differences in mortality trends between the member countries of the Council of Europe led Caselli & Egidi (*2*) to conclude, that "although there is a relationship between life span, socio-economic conditions and the standard of public health service, it is obviously not a straight-forward one". The impact of development in health, at the low levels of mortality that prevail in Europe at least, is likely to be related more to the quality of health care than to the effects of the environment itself. Moreover, the contribution from unhealthy lifestyles is likely to be of much greater consequence.

It is interesting to observe also that occasionally one can view mortality experiences from actual situations that closely resemble, in some respects at least, controlled epidemiological trials. One such example is the German Democratic Republic and the Federal Republic of Germany, which have now been through 35 years of socialist and capitalist development, respectively, based on more or less the same material and technical resources. Fig. 1 shows the trend of life expectancy at birth and at 30 years of age for men and women in these two countries. In the early 1950s life expectancy at birth was higher in the Federal Republic than in the Democratic Republic; by 1955 the levels were roughly identical for males, while for women this was achieved only some 10 years later. From about 1975 men in the Democratic Republic had a consistently higher life expectancy than their counterparts in the West, and women in both countries followed the same upward trend. However, the pattern changed again in the late 1970s when life expectancy increased substantially in the Federal Republic — 0.86 years for women from 1975–1977 to 1977–1979 — whereas life expectancy has remained constant in the Democratic Republic. That increase in life expectancy was due to a decrease in the age-specific death rates in all five-year age groups between 1975 and 1979 (*6*). It would be interesting to study causes of death contributing to these changes.

Social class differences

The social class pattern in mortality is known for only a few European countries: Denmark, England & Wales, Finland, France, Norway and Sweden. Because the social class classifications are based on occupation, reliable data for social class differences in mortality mainly exist for people in the economically active age groups. However, it has been estimated for

Fig. 1. Life expectancy at birth and at 30 years of age for men and women in the German Democratic Republic and the Federal Republic of Germany

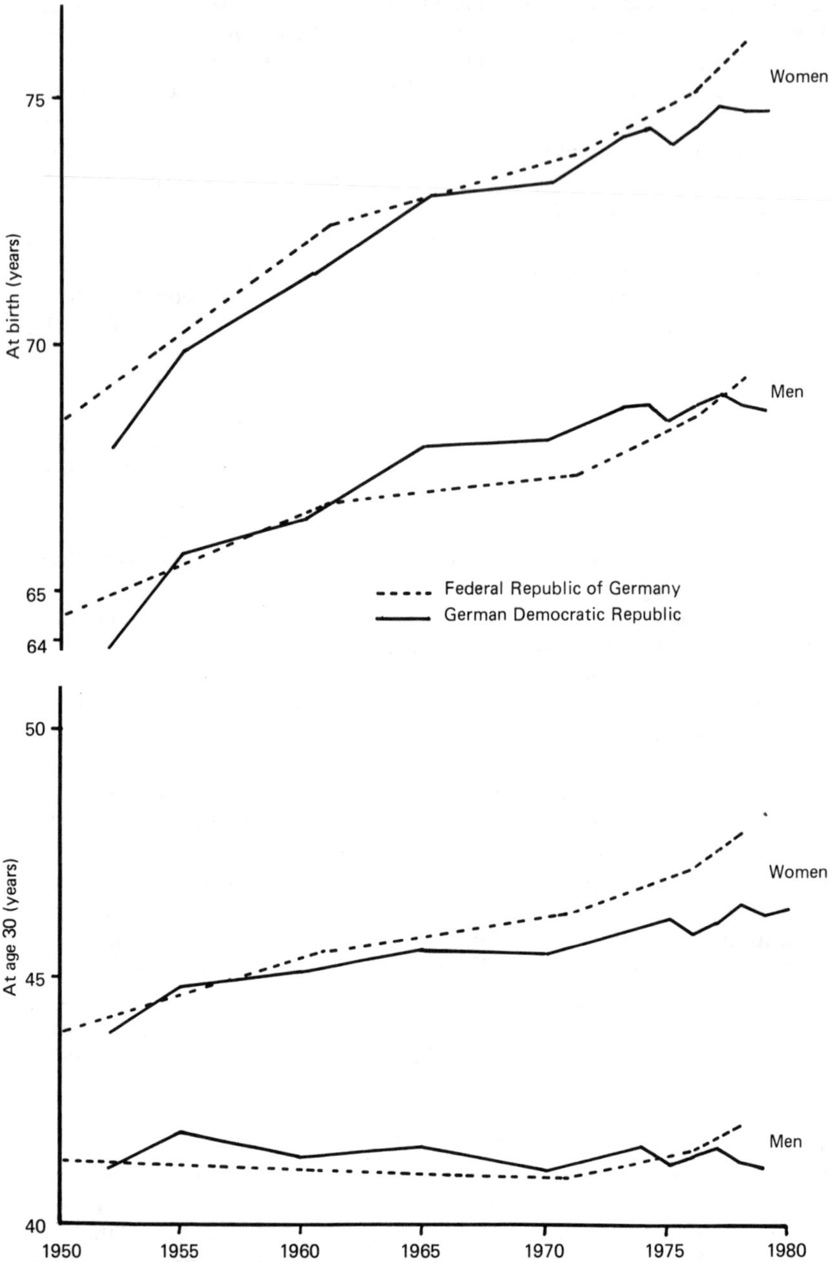

Source: (*6, 7*).

England & Wales that the life expectancy at birth is 72.19 years for males in social class I and only 65.02 years for males belonging to social class V. This estimation is based on classification of children by their fathers' social class and of men aged 15–64 years by their own social class, and on the assumption that social class I men aged over 65 have a 20% lower mortality than all men and that social class V men have 20% higher mortality (*8*). Despite its limitations, this procedure suggests that the social class difference in mortality for men in England & Wales is of the same order as that between men in Portugal and Scandinavia.

Furthermore, since a person's position in the labour market is very sensitive to his health conditions, the recorded social class difference in mortality is highly dependent on the definitions, classifications, etc. used in a study. Therefore, one has to be aware of inconsistencies in respect of these factors when data from different studies are compared. Nonetheless, it is possible to discern equal social class patterns in mortality in different countries. For instance, unskilled and semi-skilled male workers in Denmark, England & Wales, and Norway have a 40–50% excess mortality at 30–40 years of age, and in all countries the excess decreases with age (Fig. 2 and 3).

Only for the Scandinavian countries can one compare mortality among women by their occupation. The data also show social class differences, which are smaller than the differences observed for men, but more stable with age. Additionally, housewives constitute a high-risk group compared with economically active women, suggesting that unhealthy women are selected out of the labour market.

Mortality Trends in Europe

Growth in life expectancy

In evaluating trends it is important to be aware of changes in the definitions that may have occurred during the period of interest. The country report for Czechoslovakia points out that the internationally recommended definition of a "live-born fetus" was accepted in Czechoslovakia in 1965. This meant a return to the definition used until 1948, whereas more restrictive definitions had been used in the mean time. This change of definition alone implied a drop in life expectancy, from 67.76 years for men in 1964 to 67.27 years in 1965. It is therefore important in the evaluation of trends to be aware of such changes in formal definitions or in the efficiency of the reporting system.

The growth in life expectancy from 1950 or so to 1978 strongly depends on the mortality level at the beginning of the period. There has been a 7- to 8-year increase for men in countries where the life expectancy in 1950 was 60 years, but an increase of only 1–2 years in countries where the life expectancy was 70 years (e.g. Denmark, the Netherlands, Norway and Sweden). For women life expectancy has increased by 9–10 years in countries such as Spain and Yugoslavia where the initial level was 65 years, and by 7–8 years in countries where life expectancy around the middle of the century was closer to 70 years. The mortality differences in Europe are consequently smaller today than in the period immediately following the Second World War.

Fig. 2. Mortality in unskilled and semi-skilled male workers compared with that in all working men in Denmark and Norway

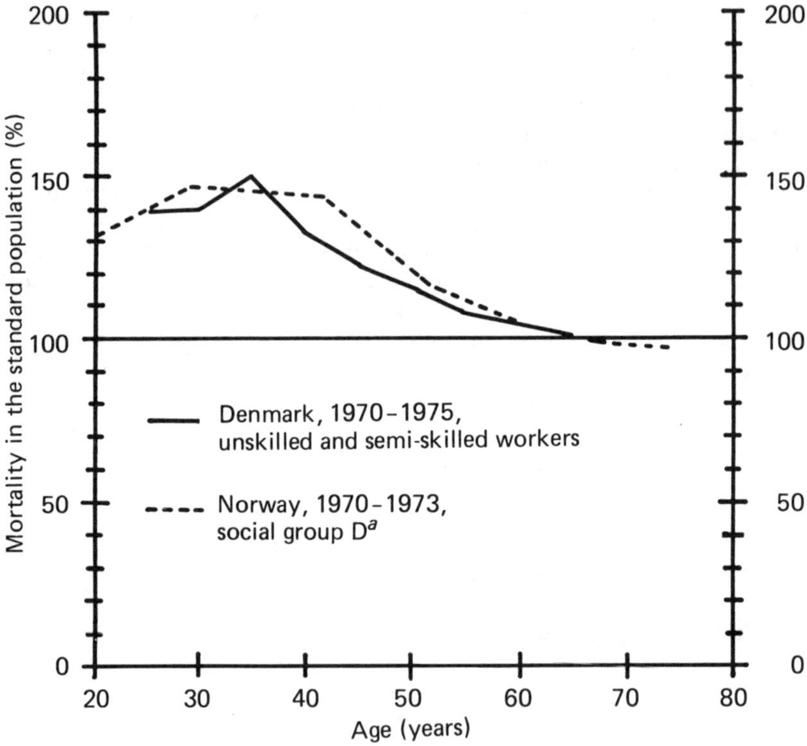

[a] Based on 1970 census.

Source: Lynge, E. & Jeune, B. (*9*).

Adverse trends

Compared with these developments, the adverse trends that have occurred over the period are perhaps less spectacular. These trends are important, however, because they indicate deteriorations in a situation where the economic and technical possibilities for further improvement are available.

The adverse trends in mortality have been observed primarily among middle-aged men. The main types of post-war trends in mortality for middle-aged men in Europe are illustrated in Fig. 4. The mortality rates for 40–69-year-old men in the Netherlands increased in the 1950s and 1960s, and although this increase ceased in the 1970s, the present level remains above that of the early 1950s. A similar pattern is seen in Denmark and

Fig. 3. Mortality in unskilled and semi-skilled male workers compared with that in all working men in England & Wales and Norway

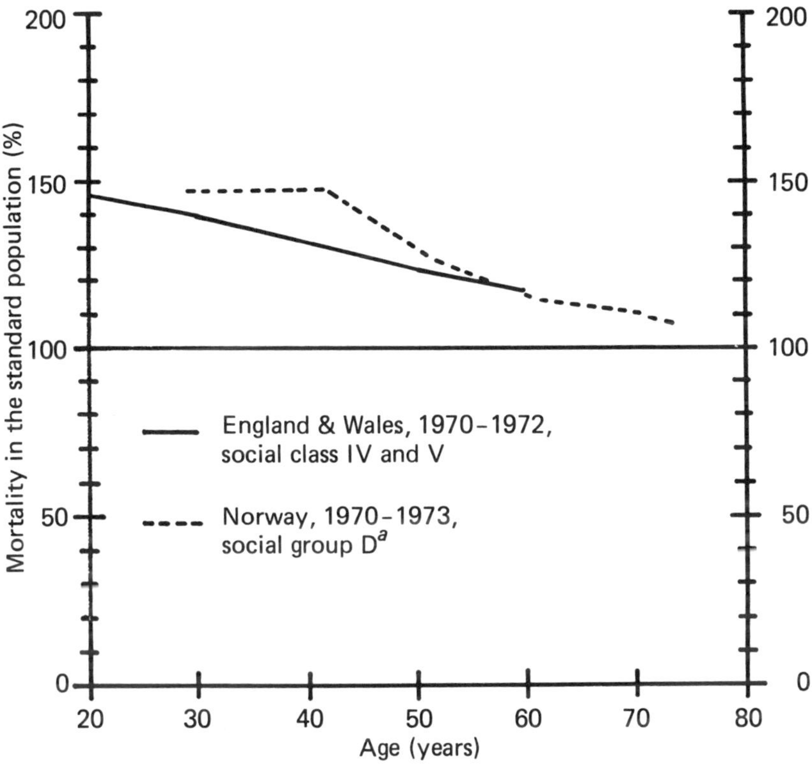

[a] Based on 1960 and 1970 censuses combined.

Source: Lynge, E. & Jeune, B. (*9*).

Norway. In England & Wales the mortality for middle-aged men declined throughout the period, but is still at a considerably higher level than in the Netherlands. A similar trend is seen in Switzerland, although at a lower level than in the United Kingdom.

Owing to an increase in the early 1950s followed by a decrease in the 1970s, the mortality for middle-aged men in the Federal Republic of Germany has remained nearly unchanged. Stable mortality for middle-aged men is also seen in Belgium, Finland, the German Democratic Republic, Portugal and Sweden, though at different levels. Adult males in Hungary up to the age of 55 years experienced a decline in mortality in the 1950s and 1960s but a steep increase in the 1970s; for men over 60 mortality increased throughout the

Fig. 4. Mortality rates for men aged 40–69 years in selected European countries, 1950–1980[a]

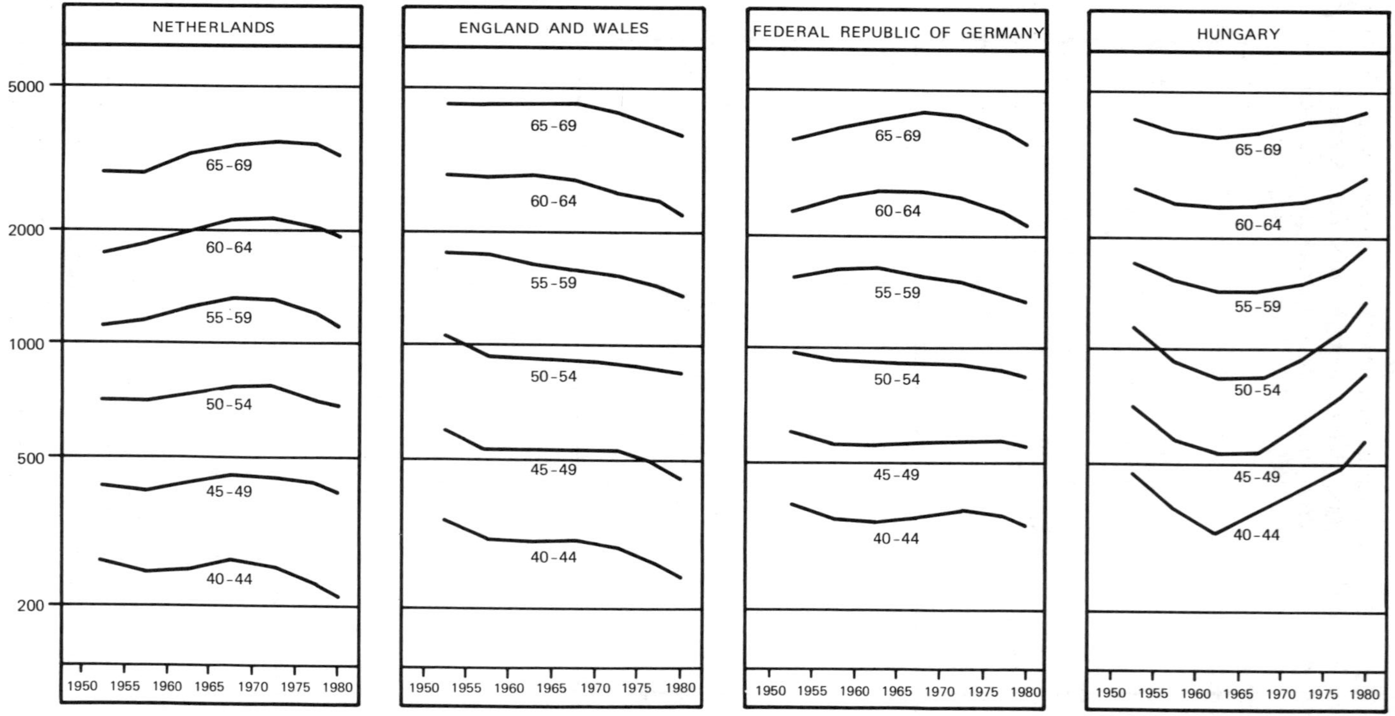

[a] Rates per 100 000 population; log scale.

post-war period. To a certain extent the same pattern is seen in Austria, Bulgaria, Czechoslovakia, Poland and Yugoslavia. In short, the predominantly adverse trends in mortality for middle-aged men have been the increase from around 1960 in some Western European countries — an increase that has now ceased — and the rise in death rates in some Eastern European countries that started at different points in time for different age groups.

From the country reports for Czechoslovakia and Norway it is possible to study the trends in main causes of death for middle-aged men over the period 1960–1979. Table 5 shows that the increase between 1960 and 1970 in the death rate for men aged 40–69 years in Czechoslovakia was mainly due to an increase in mortality from circulatory diseases. Table 6 shows that the death rate for 40–69-year-old men in Norway reached a peak in the late 1960s, and the changes here are also due mainly to circulatory diseases. Cancer mortality is increasing for middle-aged men in both countries. A similar trend can be seen for the Netherlands. Moreover, since death rates for women continued to decline, this stagnation/increase for adult males has resulted in the increased difference in life expectancy between men and women (*10*).

Table 5. Age-standardized[a] mortality rates (per 100 000) for men aged 40–69 years in Czechoslovakia, 1960–1979

Cause of death	Period			
	1960–1964	1965–1969	1970–1974	1975–1979
All causes	397	421	451	445
Circulatory diseases	123	153	195	195
Neoplasms	116	119	122	125
Respiratory diseases	35	37	38	33
Injuries and poisoning	36	39	41	39

[a] Based on the world standard population composition.

However, in recent years stagnations and increases have also been observed for women, especially around the age of 50. In Denmark death rates for women aged 45–59 have remained constant over the period from 1960–1964 to 1979, and the same pattern is seen for women in Czechoslovakia. The recent increase in mortality in Hungary has affected women aged 40–64 years.

Table 6. Age-standardized[a] mortality rates (per 100 000) for men aged 40–69 years in Norway, 1961–1979

Cause of death	Period			
	1961–1965	1966–1970	1971–1975	1976–1979
All causes	293	306	298	291
Cardiovascular diseases	142	155	150	143
Malignant neoplasms	67	68	70	74
Violent death (except suicide)	18	18	19	17
Suicide	6	6	7	7

[a] Based on the world standard population composition.

The identification and investigation of subgroups of the population that experience such adverse trends in mortality is clearly of paramount importance. Such studies may often reveal complex patterns. For example, suicide rates in men increase with decreasing social status in both Denmark and Finland, whereas the opposite is true for women (*11*). A complex social pattern would therefore appear to underlie the increasing suicide rates reported for both men and women in the Netherlands and Norway.

Trends in social class differences

Although data on socioeconomic differences in mortality are now available from several countries, only those from the United Kingdom provide the possibility for studying trends in social class differences. Fig. 5 shows the age-standardized death rates for men aged 15–64 years in social classes I and V in 1949–1953, 1959–1963 and 1970–1972 in England & Wales, adjusted in each case to the 1950 occupational classification. The social class difference increased between 1951 and 1961, but appears to have stabilized during the following decade. The different social classes have therefore been affected differently by the overall decline in mortality observed in Fig. 4 for adult men in England & Wales.

In a French study, the mortality among a sample of men from the 1954 census was followed throughout the period 1955–1971. The study indicates an increase in the mortality difference between social groups from 1955–1960 to 1966–1971; but due to the follow-up design of the study the data are influenced by the so-called "healthy worker effect" and are therefore difficult to interpret (*11*).

Fig. 5. Trends in death rates for men aged 15–64 years in social classes I and V, England & Wales, 1951–1971

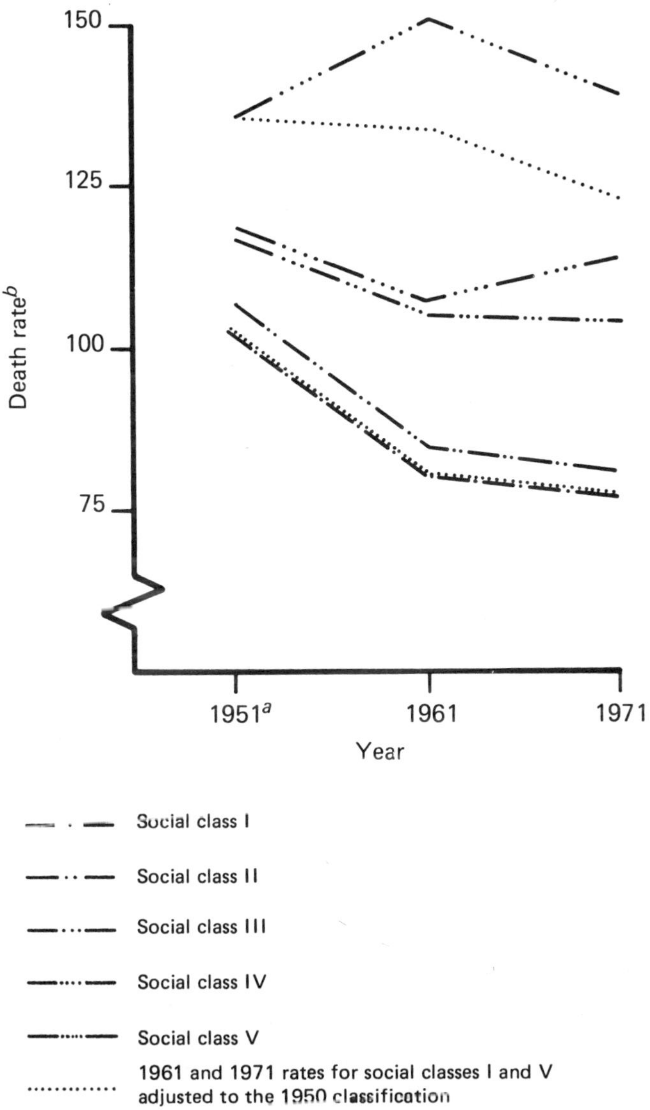

[a] 1951 rates were adjusted for errors and changes to social class IV.

[b] Direct age-standardized death rate per 100 000 living at ages 15–64 using all men in 1970–1972 as the standard.

Source: Office of Population Censuses and Surveys (*8*).

Conclusions and Implications for Health and Social Policy

From the health policy point of view the adverse trends in mortality are the most important to concentrate on. The adverse trends so far seen have almost solely affected men; the main cause of death has been circulatory diseases, and social class differences in mortality seem to have increased simultaneously. Cigarette smoking, higher calorific intake and mechanization of industry and transport are probably the main causes behind these adverse trends (*10*). Identification of the causes behind the increase in mortality *and* behind the subsequent decrease in certain European countries is important in order to control possible deterioration. Trends in female mortality should also be monitored closely.

The widening of the gap between men and women in life expectancy will highly influence the sex composition of older age groups. Given a sex difference in life expectancy of 5–10 years, and the fact that women tend to marry older men, women can now expect to live on average 10–15 years in widowhood. Maintenance of social networks for elderly women therefore seems to be an important task from the social policy point of view.

References

1. **McKeown, T. & Record, R.G.** Reasons for the decline in mortality in England & Wales during the nineteenth century. *Population studies,* **16**: 94 (1962).
2. **Caselli, G. & Egidi, V.** *New trends in European mortality.* Strasbourg, Council of Europe, 1980.
3. *World health statistics annual, 1980.* Geneva, World Health Organization, 1980.
4. *Demographic yearbook, 1979.* New York, United Nations, 1980.
5. *Nordic yearbook of statistics, 1980.* Stockholm, Nordic Statistical Secretariat, 1981.
6. *Statistisches Jahrbuch 1979 und 1981 für die BRD.*
7. *Statistisches Jahrbuch 1979 und 1981 der DDR.*
8. **Office of Population Censuses and Surveys.** *Occupational mortality 1970–72. England and Wales. Decennial supplement.* London, H.M. Stationery Office, 1978.
9. **Lynge, E. & Jeune, B.** Excess mortality among male unskilled and semi-skilled workers. *Scandinavian journal of social medicine,* **11**: 37–40 (1983).
10. **Lopez, A.D.** The changing sex mortality differential in developed countries. *In:* Lopez, A.D. & Ruzicka, L.T., ed. *Sex differentials in mortality: trends, determinants and consequences.* Canberra, Australian National University Press, 1983.
11. **Lynge, E.** *Socio-economic differences in mortality in Europe.* Strasbourg, Council of Europe, 1983.

Part III

Health and social implications

5

Implications of demographic change for the young population (0–19 years)

S. Teper & M. Backett

The demographic changes that are taking place in the European Region are, in some respects, of a type that has not previously occurred. Good social policies will be those that are ready to reflect an anticipated response to these changes. The difficulty, as with most aspects of the human ecosystem, is that once the details of change are considered, there are often many variables and so little is certain.

What is known for sure is that the social (in the broadest sense of the term) and economic repercussions of the population change that is already in train are likely to be immense, and careful consideration must be given to selecting those policies that are most likely to lead to societal and individual health and happiness.

That this is more easily said than done can be seen from the nature of the available data, consisting of few facts (or even supported inferences) and many speculations, and from the large number of groups in the population who are likely to be vulnerable.

This chapter focuses on those under 20 years of age — arguably the most important group of all in society, and probably the group about which the least is known in relation to health or other areas of life. This is despite the fact that the determinants of later health and behaviour are laid down at these ages. Family influences and education are of the highest importance, and these give way to the development of peer group pressures. These experiences ultimately influence patterns of assortative mating, occupational skills and the extremes of belief. The childhood years are the period in which the transmission of attitudes and behaviour, the so-called "socialization process", is probably of vital importance in relation to many aspects of adult life — aspects as widely different as, for example, the later genesis of chronic disease and the determinants of political attitudes (*1,2*). As the very young reach adulthood, the huge impact of changes in lifestyle and in health can be seen.

Aspects of Population Change

The latest world population projections (medium variant) from the United Nations suggest that the total population of the European Region of the

World Health Organization will increase by 16.7% between 1980 and the year 2000; this implies an average annual rate of growth of about 0.8% (*3*). Using the United Nations geographical divisions of Europe, it is clear that population growth will vary between these divisions (Table 1). When the population growth in individual countries is examined, we can see that very real variations also exist. Two countries will experience a decline in population numbers, several other countries will experience just a very small increase and others will have relatively high rates of growth. A fourth group of countries will experience massive population growth (Table 1).

Changes in the size of population groups in Europe, with special reference to those aged under 20 years

Even with relatively stable total numbers in the population, significant numerical change can take place in the size of each major age group (the major age groups have been taken as 0–19, 20–59 and 60 years and over). In addition, the impact of demographic change can be radically different from one age group to another. The first three columns of Table 1 illustrate this point.

Sixteen of the countries listed in Table 1 will experience a decline in the numbers aged under 20 years; in four cases (Austria, the German Democratic Republic, the Federal Republic of Germany and Switzerland) the decline is greater than 10%. A further nine countries will experience no change or a slight increase — of at most 7% — in the number of young people. Three countries show a more substantial increase: Albania (nearly 11%), Czechoslovakia (9%) and the USSR (10.5%). In the remaining three countries — Algeria, Morocco and Turkey — the numbers in this age group will become very much larger by the end of the century (by 81%, 58% and 33% respectively).

When the four contiguous European subregions are considered (i.e. excluding Algeria, Morocco, Turkey and the USSR) it is only in Eastern Europe than an overall increase (3%) in young people will be seen; in the other three areas an overall decrease is evident.

It should be noted, however, that in some countries the numbers of young people will increase before they start to decline, as a function of the size of previous birth cohorts. In other countries there will be a steady decline until almost the end of the century, when the numbers will rise slightly, reflecting larger birth cohorts from increasing numbers of women likely to have children.

Although changes at both ends of the age spectrum are likely to have a significant impact on individual societies, columns 2 and 3 of Table 1 demonstrate quite explicitly that the changes in the two older age groups will be far larger. This statement applies particularly to the age group 60 years and over. The social and economic implications of the changes in the retired population (and to a slightly lesser extent in the working age group) are so dramatic and demanding that they may well take priority over the needs of the young.

Another important aspect of structural adjustment to population change is whether or not the pattern of change in the period 1980–2000 is a

Table 1. Percentage changes in the absolute numbers in the major age groups between 1980 and 2000 in the countries of the WHO European Region

Region and country	Age group			
	0–19	20–59	60+	All ages
Eastern Europe	+ 3.2	+ 8.8	+32.9	+10.7
Bulgaria	+ 2.0	+ 1.0	+41.7	+ 7.7
Czechoslovakia	+ 9.0	+ 12.6	+16.8	+12.1
German Democratic Republic[a]	- 15.7	+ 3.6	+ 9.3	- 0.7
Hungary	+ 3.1	+ 0.7	+19.8	+ 4.6
Poland	+ 6.7	+ 12.7	+45.7	+15.1
Romania	+ 6.7	+ 10.8	+56.1	+15.5
Northern Europe[b]	- 6.8	+ 9.4	+ 1.9	+ 3.2
Denmark	- 6.4	+ 8.9	+ 4.1	+ 3.6
Finland	- 2.6	+ 6.7	+19.1	+ 6.1
Iceland[c]	- 2.4	+ 33.0	+33.3	+19.9
Ireland	+ 1.2	+ 46.3	+ 2.4	+21.2
Norway	- 1.8	+ 17.5	- 1.1	+ 8.0
Sweden	- 2.6	+ 7.9	- 2.0	+ 3.0
United Kingdom	- 8.8	+ 7.3	+ 1.3	+ 1.4
Southern Europe[d]	- 3.2	+ 13.1	+42.7	+12.4
Albania	+10.8	+ 70.8	+91.1	+43.1
Greece	+ 3.6	+ 7.5	+36.2	+11.4
Italy	- 7.6	+ 6.3	+34.0	+ 7.1
Malta[c]	0	+ 15.8	+28.0	+13.8
Portugal	+ 0.3	+ 23.8	+29.9	+16.3
Spain	- 2.6	+ 20.3	+44.5	+16.0
Yugoslavia	- 1.3	+ 11.1	+77.2	+14.8
Western Europe[e]	- 7.9	+ 4.5	+17.6	+ 3.3
Austria	- 10.9	+ 7.3	+ 5.7	+ 1.8
Belgium	+ 2.6	+ 9.4	+15.1	+ 8.5
France	- 3.4	+ 9.6	+18.4	+ 7.2
Federal Republic of Germany[a]	- 13.8	- 3.2	+17.2	- 2.2
Luxembourg[c]	- 6.5	- 3.4	+23.1	+ 0.8
Netherlands	- 7.1	+ 15.7	+24.6	+10.0
Switzerland	- 10.7	+ 2.5	+20.1	+ 2.0
South-West Asia				
Turkey	+32.7	+ 70.1	+94.2	+53.1
North Africa				
Algeria	+81.0	+118.4	+65.0	+93.7
Morocco	+57.9	+106.6	+95.2	+78.1
USSR	+10.5	+ 11.2	+56.9	+16.9
WHO European Region	+ 9.5	+ 15.8	+36.2	+16.7
WHO European Region, less USSR	+ 9.1	+ 18.1	+27.9	+16.6

[a] The figures for the German Democratic Republic and the Federal Republic of Germany include the relevant data for Berlin.

[b] Includes the Channel Islands, the Faeroe Islands and the Isle of Man.

[c] Small numbers were involved in these computations.

[d] Includes Andorra, Gibraltar, The Holy See and San Marino.

[e] Includes Liechtenstein and Monaco.

Source: United Nations (*3*).

continuation of that seen in the immediately preceding period. Data illustrating this point, for those aged under 20 only, are presented in Table 2 (the right-hand column of this table is identical to the first column of Table 1). Table 2 shows that each of the four subregions has seen an overall reversal of change in the size of the number of young people. All possible combinations of increase/decrease are, however, seen amongst individual countries.

A further point to be made is that Algeria, Morocco and Turkey account, quite disproportionately, for the bulk of the increase in the under-20 age group in both periods, 1960–1980 and 1980–2000, and particularly so in the second (see Table 3).

Finally, in this section, data are presented that allow population change in those aged under 20 to be seen in a more traditional framework. Table 4 shows the percentage of the total population in this age group in each European country in 1960, 1980 and 2000. Each country within the four subregions shows a continuing reduction in the proportion of people under 20 from 1960 through to 2000. The pattern in the USSR is similar; in Algeria, Morocco and Turkey, however, a much higher proportion of the population is young — between 50% and 58% in 1980, reducing to 43–55% by 2000. Both Algeria and Morocco experienced an increase in this proportion between 1960 and 1980.

Urbanization

An important demographic topic for consideration is that of continuing urbanization in Europe. As the data for individual countries were not available, figures on the percentages living in urban areas presented in Table 5 refer to the four subregions of Europe (Algeria, Morocco, Turkey and the USSR again being excluded). The data are presented for 1975 and the year 2000, and are given by major age group and by sex. Between 1975 and the end of the century the proportion of the population living in urban areas will increase from 66% to 77%. The degree of urbanization varies by subregion of residence and by age and sex (Table 5).

A taxonomy of European countries

Demographically, Europe is often assumed to be a relatively homogeneous unit yet, as shown above, population change over the next 20 years will have a markedly different impact on individual countries. Use of the United Nations definition of European subregions (which has been done for simplicity in presenting the tabular material so far) in a way is not of great assistance in predicting and interpreting the social effect of population change, since variations within the subregions are real and large. For the purpose of looking in a practical way at the implications of demographic change for social, economic and health policy, it would be useful to have a taxonomy of countries. This would enable one to deal with a few groups of countries, within each of which the demographic impact of population change is likely to be broadly similar, rather than to continue dealing with the traditional (basically geographic) divisions of the Region, or with individual countries. Such a taxonomy could have been developed on an economic basis, in terms of cultural variables or in relation to the likely political

Table 2. Percentage changes in the absolute numbers in the population aged 0–19 years, 1960–1980 and 1980–2000, in the countries of the WHO European Region

Region and country	Percentage change during:	
	1960–1980	1980–2000
Eastern Europe	- 0.6	+ 3.2
Bulgaria	- 1.0	+ 2.0
Czechoslovakia	- 0.4	+ 9.0
German Democratic Republic[a]	- 3.5	- 15.7
Hungary	- 9.5	+ 3.1
Poland	- 3.8	+ 6.7
Romania	+12.0	+ 6.7
Northern Europe[b]	+ 1.4	- 6.8
Denmark	- 5.1	- 6.4
Finland	- 19.5	- 2.6
Iceland[c]	+13.3	- 2.4
Ireland	+19.7	+ 1.2
Norway	+ 2.6	- 1.8
Sweden	- 1.8	- 2.6
United Kingdom	+ 3.2	- 8.8
Southern Europe[d]	+ 9.4	- 3.2
Albania	+59.7	+10.8
Greece	+ 0.2	+ 3.6
Italy	+ 4.7	- 7.6
Malta[c]	- 28.7	0
Portugal	+ 5.7	+ 0.3
Spain	+20.4	- 2.6
Yugoslavia	+ 3.7	- 1.3
Western Europe[e]	+ 5.2	- 7.9
Austria	+ 2.5	- 10.9
Belgium	+ 5.0	+ 2.6
France	+ 9.1	- 3.4
Federal Republic of Germany[a]	+ 3.3	- 13.8
Luxembourg[c]	+ 5.7	- 6.5
Netherlands	+ 0.6	- 7.1
Switzerland	+ 3.2	- 10.7
South-West Asia		
Turkey	+65.1	+32.7
North Africa		
Algeria	+88.1	+81.0
Morocco	+81.2	+57.9
USSR	+13.3	+10.5
WHO European Region	+14.6	+ 9.5
WHO European Region, less USSR	+15.2	+ 9.1

[a] The figures for the German Democratic Republic and the Federal Republic of Germany include the relevant data for Berlin.

[b] Includes the Channel Islands, the Faeroe Islands and the Isle of Man.

[c] Small numbers were involved in these computations.

[d] Includes Andorra, Gibraltar, The Holy See and San Marino.

[e] Includes Liechtenstein and Monaco.

Source: United Nations (*3*).

Table 3. Numerical changes in the absolute numbers in the population aged 0–19 years, 1960–1980 and 1980–2000, in groups of European countries

Country group	Year	Total population aged 0–19 years	Increase/decrease during:	
			1960–1980	1980–2000
Eastern, Northern, Southern and Western Europe	1980 2000	140 459 141 137	+ 6 152	- 5 474
Algeria, Morocco and Turkey	1980 2000	25 856 67 979	+19 190	+22 933
USSR	1980 2000	78 894 98 801	+10 531	- 9 376
WHO European Region	1980 2000	245 209 307 917	+35 873	+26 835

Source: United Nations (*3*).

response to change. However, since this book deals very specifically with the impact of population change, it was felt that the taxonomy should have a fundamental demographic basis.

Societal resources can be viewed as elements for which individual population groups compete. Whatever the real needs of the young, what is actually made available to them over the next two decades will reflect the broader economic and social adjustments that are essential if an attempt is to be made to cope with the massive changes in the adult population. Accordingly, the other basic facet of the taxonomy is that it considers the balance of population change within a country, not merely trends among those under 20 years of age.

The basic data for developing the taxonomy are those presented in Table 1. The first stage, for each individual country, was to classify each of the two older major age groups in terms of whether they will experience what has been termed "little growth" or "high growth" in absolute numbers between 1980 and the end of the century. For those under 20 three categories were used: a marked decline in numbers, little change and high growth. The cut-off points for each category were derived on the basis of the total population of Europe according to the United Nations classification, and were fixed at the following intervals: –15.7% to –6.4%, –3.4% to +3.1%, and 6.7% or more. Algeria, Morocco and Turkey were not included since their demographic structures differ so radically from most of the rest of Europe; the USSR was also not included because its relatively large numbers would have swamped the whole taxonomy. The cut-off points are set crudely at the mean United Nations figures for change in Europe between 1980 and the year 2000.

Table 4. Those aged 0–19 years as a percentage of the total population in 1960, 1980 and 2000, in countries of the WHO European Region

Region and country	Percentage of total population in:		
	1960	1980	2000
Eastern Europe	35.1	30.7	28.6
Bulgaria	33.6	29.0	27.5
Czechoslovakia	35.1	31.1	30.3
German Democratic Republic[a]	28.3	27.9	23.7
Hungary	32.8	27.6	27.2
Poland	40.1	31.8	29.5
Romania	35.5	32.9	30.4
Northern Europe[b]	31.3	29.4	26.5
Denmark	33.6	28.6	25.8
Finland	38.5	28.5	26.1
Iceland[c]	42.6	36.8	30.0
Ireland	39.4	40.4	33.7
Norway	33.2	29.9	27.2
Sweden	29.9	26.6	25.2
United Kingdom	30.1	29.2	26.3
Southern Europe[d]	34.8	32.3	27.8
Albania	50.8	48.6	37.7
Greece	34.0	30.4	28.3
Italy	32.2	29.7	25.6
Malta[c]	45.0	31.5	27.6
Portugal	37.5	35.6	30.7
Spain	35.4	34.5	29.0
Yugoslavia	38.3	32.7	28.1
Western Europe[e]	31.0	28.7	25.6
Austria	30.0	29.0	25.4
Belgium	29.5	28.6	27.0
France	32.5	30.3	27.3
Federal Republic of Germany[a]	28.7	26.9	23.8
Luxembourg[c]	27.7	25.7	23.8
Netherlands	37.9	31.1	26.3
Switzerland	31.5	27.6	24.1
South-West Asia			
Turkey	49.6	49.6	43.0
North Africa			
Algeria	53.6	58.6	54.7
Morocco	55.3	57.4	50.9
USSR	36.8	33.5	31.7
WHO European Region	35.6	33.7	31.6
WHO European Region, less USSR	35.0	33.8	31.6

[a] The figures for the German Democratic Republic and the Federal Republic of Germany include the relevant data for Berlin

[b] Includes the Channel Islands, the Faeroe Islands and the Isle of Man.

[c] Small numbers were involved in these computations.

[d] Includes Andorra, Gibraltar, The Holy See and San Marino.

[e] Includes Liechtenstein and Monaco.

Source: United Nations (*3*).

Table 5. Percentages of the population living in urban areas in 1975 and 2000, by major age group and sex

Region	Age group (years)							
	0–19		20–59		60+		All ages	
	1975	2000	1975	2000	1975	2000	1975	2000
Both sexes								
All Europe	62.7	73.9	68.8	79.5	66.7	75.7	66.4	77.1
Eastern Europe	52.9	67.3	59.0	73.6	53.8	66.5	56.2	70.5
Northern Europe	82.0	89.1	84.3	90.7	83.6	89.7	83.4	89.6
Southern Europe	53.2	67.7	59.4	73.2	53.3	66.9	56.2	70.3
Western Europe	72.9	81.0	78.1	86.0	76.7	84.4	76.3	84.3
Males								
All Europe	62.8	74.0	68.5	79.4	63.7	73.3	65.8	76.8
Eastern Europe	52.8	67.2	58.7	73.4	51.1	64.2	55.6	70.1
Northern Europe	81.7	88.7	83.5	89.9	80.0	86.9	82.5	89.1
Southern Europe	53.6	68.2	59.5	73.8	50.8	64.5	56.1	70.5
Western Europe	72.7	80.8	77.3	85.2	73.8	82.0	75.3	83.4
Females								
All Europe	62.7	73.8	69.1	79.7	68.9	77.7	67.0	77.5
Eastern Europe	53.0	67.5	59.3	73.9	55.8	68.2	56.8	70.9
Northern Europe	82.4	89.4	85.1	91.5	85.6	91.7	84.4	91.0
Southern Europe	52.8	67.1	59.3	72.6	55.2	68.7	56.3	70.1
Western Europe	73.1	81.2	78.9	86.8	78.8	86.4	77.2	85.2

Source: United Nations (*3*).

Having classified the population groups in this way, the countries constituting the WHO European Region fell into four broad categories, as described in Table 6.

The basic data used earlier in this chapter are also presented in Table 6 according to this taxonomy, along with the growth patterns for the separate country groups. This revised presentation of the data suggests that only in category A countries are societal priorities likely to be decided by broad social preferences and not dictated by demography. In categories B, and particularly C, policy is unlikely to be orientated towards the young. To a lesser extent this last statement also applies to the remaining six countries in category D. The structure of Table 6 should stand as a framework against which to interpret the discussion section that follows.

Table 6. Countries of the WHO European Region classified by growth in absolute numbers between 1980 and 2000

Category	Percentage absolute change in each age group 0–19	20–59	60+	All ages	Total population in 1980 (millions)
A (12 countries)					
Little growth in all three age groups; some countries have a decline in those aged under 20	*- 8.0*	*+ 4.5*	*+11.6*	*+ 2.3*	*240.1*
Five countries with little change in those aged under 20 (Belgium, Finland, France, Hungary, Sweden)	- 1.9	+ 8.1	+15.8	+ 6.5	87.2
Seven countries with a marked decline in those aged under 20 (Austria, Denmark, German Dem. Rep., Fed. Rep. of Germany, Luxembourg, Switzerland, UK)	- 11.6	+ 2.4	+ 9.4	- 0.2	152.9
B (5 countries)					
Little growth in those aged under 20; high growth in the age groups 20–59 and 60 years and over (Iceland, Malta, Portugal, Spain, Yugoslavia)	*- 1.8*	*+17.6*	*+51.1*	*+15.7*	*70.1*
C (8 countries, including the USSR)					
High growth in all three major age groups	*+21.4*	*+23.8*	*+57.1*	*+26.8*	*427.0*
(Albania, Algeria, Czechoslovakia[a], Morocco, Poland, Romania, Turkey)	+35.4	+47.5	+57.4	+43.2	160.4
(USSR)	+10.5	+11.5	+56.9	+16.9	266.7
D (6 countries)					
Residual countries with little change or a decline in those aged under 20, and high growth in one only of the two other age groups	*- 4.9*	*+ 8.9*	*+31.3*	*+ 8.5*	*96.8*
Three countries with high growth in the 20-59 age group (Ireland, Netherlands, Norway)	- 4.6	+20.1	+15.4	+11.3	75.3
Three countries with high growth in the 60+ age group (Bulgaria, Greece, Italy)	- 5.1	+ 5.7	+35.6	+ 7.7	21.5
WHO European Region	*+ 9.5*	*+15.8*	*+36.2*	*+16.7*	
WHO European Region, less USSR	+ 9.1	+18.1	+27.9	+16.6	
Europe, United Nations definition[b]	- 3.7	+ 8.8	+24.3	+ 7.6	

[a] Czechoslovakia is placed in this category because it is unique among these countries in having high growth in the under-20 and 20–59-year age groups, but lower growth in the retired population. See Table 1.

[b] Used in determining the basic taxonomy (see text).

Demographic Events in the Under-20 Age Group

Although the discussion to this point has focused on the effects of demographic change on young people against the broader aspects of population change, it is important to remember that this age group is itself subject to demographic events. In particular, its number and structure may be affected by mortality, migration, marriage and parenthood.

The projections provided by the United Nations imply improving expectation of life at birth; this improvement is made up of lower age-specific mortality together with improved infant survival. In Europe we can anticipate improvements in obstetric and neonatal knowledge, technology and care over the next 20 years. Thus, more of the babies who will be born between now and the end of the century will survive to adulthood. More handicapped babies, and more small children damaged by accidents or by disease, will also survive. In relation to specific causes of morbidity and mortality at young ages — particularly among males — mention should also be made of accidents in general, and road traffic accidents in particular (*4,5*).

Those countries within the WHO European Region that comprise the main part of the European Community can expect some employment-related migration, given the Community regulations in that respect. The present world economic situation may, however, make such movements possible more in theory than in practice. As noted earlier, migration in terms of urbanization will continue until the end of the period under consideration.

In many countries, marriage before the age of 20 has become increasingly popular. Such marriages, however, are more likely than others to end in divorce, and they are also often associated with premarital pregnancy (*6–10*). Marriage (and parenthood) when very young affects future life opportunities for the young adults involved, particularly so for women. Although there is no way one can predict marriage patterns among young people in Europe over the next two decades, there is increasing evidence both of premarital cohabitation and of cohabitation as an alternative to marriage (*11–13*). Whether this will have an effect on ultimate patterns of marriage and/or childbearing remains quite unknown. These statements on premarital cohabitation and pregnancy do not apply to all the countries of Europe. In some countries the traditional pattern of chaperoning restricts the social and sexual association of young people. In other countries early marriage prevents premarital cohabitation and pregnancy; for example, data from Algeria indicate that 31% of women who marry do so before the age of 15 and 72% before the age of 20 (*14*).

Although there has been considerable study of the relationship between divorce and fertility, little is as yet known about the effect of parental divorce (and remarriage) on the children — that is, on the young people whom we are considering in this chapter. On the whole, the present generation of children and young adults is the first to have experienced parental divorce on a large scale. Another unknown factor is what the effect will be of present family size on future reproductive patterns. Data from the World Fertility Survey show that recent total fertility rates for 11 European countries have reached unprecedentedly low levels — on average, the young during the remainder of this century will have been born into small families (see Chapter 2). There is one final point to be made in relation to marriage and divorce among those under 20 years of age. This is that the *excess* supply of males may mean that the age differences between partners could increase for at least a proportion of couples marrying. Furthermore, depending on the age pattern of divorce, remarriage may be relatively more difficult for men than for women, a reverse of the situation in the recent past.

The Needs of the Under-20 Age Group

Just as the nature of population patterns becomes more speculative as demographic projections reach further into the future, so estimates of the needs of the people concerned must become increasingly speculative. However, it is upon such speculations that social policies must be built. There is no real alternative: either policies anticipate the changes that are pending or, as so often in history, they are too little and too late. The notion of anticipatory social policy as "good" policy carries with it the implication that a society must seek to meet at least the basic needs of its populations; they must be fed, clothed, housed, educated, employed and rewarded, their health must be protected, and their security, happiness and chosen lifestyles must be promoted. The building and planning of families must be facilitated and their standards of living (including their creative, cultural and religious standards) maintained so that they conform to societal aspirations.

Unfortunately there are two difficulties in such a formulation. First, it is too paternalistic by far: the society that is conceived in these terms is (or should be) making its own policies, and the very act of participation in policy formulation for the common good may meet a profound social and psychological need. Second, it is far too simplistic to see demographic structure as the starting point in an analysis of social, economic and other effects. It is much more likely that one is here dealing with an interacting system to which a systems approach is more appropriate.

Given the probable demographic trends within the European Region it is possible to guess not only which are likely to be the most sensitive or vulnerable groups — that is, those population groups exposed to the greatest risk that their basic needs will not be met, and for whom population structure contributes to that risk — but also to guess the likely unmet needs themselves. In addition, of course, young people are vulnerable by virtue of their age, sex, culture, place of living, socioeconomic status and a host of other variables which are only slightly affected by population structure, yet which interact with it. The two cannot easily be separated.

Needs in general

Because a relatively high standard of living is enjoyed in most of the European Region, most of the basic needs for food, clothing, etc. mentioned above are met,[a] and vulnerability springs only rarely from dire poverty,

[a] This is not so often the case in Turkey or the Mediterranean littoral.

severe malnutrition, or an absence of any health care, as it so often does in the developing world. The under-20 age group in the European cultures is, however, especially vulnerable in certain psychosocial fields, in some health matters, to unemployment, to the strident emphasis on inequalities by the media, and to the anomie associated with affluent urban societies. All this is well known, and there is an abundant literature that stresses in addition the special vulnerability of the new waves of migrants (only a few of whom are in this age group), those who drift to the cities, the loners and the lonely, the unemployed (perhaps a particularly serious assault on the adolescent), the parentless and, of course, some special groups such as pregnant unmarried teenage girls.

However, in all parts of the Region those under 20 have never been so healthy physically. The increasing biological gap between puberty and adulthood, which lengthens the "equivocal and uncertain" period of adolescence, together with the retreat of infectious disease, leaves accidents as the main health hazard to this group. While the dangerous home and the motor vehicle threaten the toddler, the geographic dispersal of friends and family and the lightweight motorcycle conspire to make adolescence the most vulnerable age within this group (*15–17*). Other health hazards to the under-20 group in the European Region are, of course, some perinatal death and congenital abnormality and the childhood cancers, which make a considerable proportionate contribution to the declining death rates (*18,19*). In addition, the addictive drugs, smoking, alcohol and sexually transmitted diseases are probably assuming greater importance as the tide of morbidity declines. Non-accidental violence is also increasing (*20*).

Economic needs must attempt to bridge the gap between aspirations and reality through useful employment. They must also deal with the bewildering effects of technical advance. Educational needs increase rapidly with the mushrooming technical complexity of modern industrial society, and the gap between the highly and the poorly educated widens — thus increasing the psychosocial stress on individuals. For many, a traditional education has become almost a handicap in the face of rapid technological progress.

Less easily studied, and therefore less well reported in the literature, are the probably vitally important needs for psychological support in the under-20 age group. Social and other support services for this population group may be nonexistent; when they do exist they are more often than not inappropriate. The family as the vehicle of socialization and as the source of later health behaviour (as well as the source of later chronic organic and psychological illness), the integrity of affection ties, the assurance of parental love, the notion of and effects of a participatory lifestyle, non-authoritarian schooling, and peer group membership have all been studied (*21–24*), and shown to be of fundamental importance to mental and social health. It is here that positive individual action in relation to sexual behaviour, successful parenthood, family building and preventive medicine has its origins, and it is here that the effects of demographic change can be seen in their most subtle — and frequently little reported and poorly understood — forms.

Needs and demographic trends

Research, particularly studies of cohorts of children growing up, has stressed the early years as formative in a far wider and more important sense than did the social research of the 1940s and 1950s. The emphasis has changed from a consideration of the importance of meeting basic needs to treating this period as the one in which the genesis of later chronic disease and health behaviour in general is located. Citizenship, participation, authoritarianism, peer group support, socialization, the integrity of the family, reward, employment, preventive medicine, and self-care are some of the new key words; in short, the under-20 period is more likely than ever to be subject to disturbance, and some of these disturbances are reflections of changes in population structure.

Resources and Priorities

From this brief review it is clear that priorities for social policy for the young between now and the end of the century must be focused on meeting more than the traditional basic needs. As these needs for food, clothing, etc. are met the more subtle and less well-documented needs are encountered, and estimates of priorities among these must be made. Policies to meet the needs of those under 20 will, therefore, be different for different countries but, for the sake of discussion a number of personal guesses (based as far as possible on the above schema) can be made so that the effects of demographic change may be considered. For example, the following guesses may be made.

- The problems of young people are now seen to be much more important subjects for social policy than they were previously.

- The physical health of the young is, with some exceptions, so good that health policy must shift more to the psychosocial and preventive areas. This is not the case in category C populations, where both physical and psychosocial health probably have equal priority.

- The education of the family as the vehicle for health knowledge and behaviour is now seen to be very important. Social policies should facilitate this, since family breakdown threatens it.

- Accidents, cancers, drug abuse, smoking, unwanted pregnancy and sexually transmitted diseases are likely to be no more important to the young than the psychological effects of unemployment, family breakdown, loneliness, migration, etc. The economics of youth employment are therefore a high priority in all areas.

- Biological education and family knowledge that encourage planned families and planned family building are part of good preventive medicine. Social policies to promote this sometimes conflict with existing policies or are affected by other demographically dictated priorities.

- The great increase in the number of the aged in the populations of the Region (particularly in category B, C and D countries) will conflict with attention to the young. There is evidence that the young are particularly good at coping with the elderly, and where a service role is possible policies might facilitate such service.

- Economic policies aimed at combating the drift to the cities have not been successful. Participation in decision-making and, where possible, local rewarding employment would go some way to combating the loneliness and anomie that has been reported, as well as lengthening adolescence.

While the above examples of speculative policy priorities — each of which is likely to be affected by demographic change — are mere guesswork, it is possible to be much more certain about a few demographically sensitive priority areas for health and social policy. These are:

- — the necessary shift of emphasis from physical health to mental and social health of the young;
- — the necessary emphasis on the family, its educational role and its preventive medical role;
- — the necessary emphasis on creative and rewarding employment or higher education for the young, preferably near home;
- — the necessary emphasis on an earlier adult role — especially in decision-making — for the young and their role in caring for the elderly, for those without parents, for migrants and for the handicapped;
- — the necessary emphasis on the need for more factual information as a basis for social policy-making;
- — the necessary emphasis on urgent training of personnel and the very unlikely ability of countries to achieve this; and
- — in view of the history of social policy change in the Region, the very small likelihood indeed of the needs of the young being met within the next 20 years.

References

1. **Falkner, F.** *Prevention in childhood of health problems in adult life.* Geneva, World Health Organization, 1980.
2. **Kandel, D.B., ed.** *Longitudinal research in drug use: empirical findings and methodological issues.* Washington, DC, Hemisphere, 1978.
3. *World population and its age-sex composition by country, 1950–2000: demographic estimation and projection as assessed in 1978.* New York, United Nations, 1980.
4. Accidents in general practice. (Editorial.) *New Zealand medical journal,* **87**: 48–49 (1978).
5. **Jeanneret, O. & Frutigen, P.** Accidents in children: the potential contribution of the paediatrician to the field research approach. *Paediatrician,* **9**: 358–367 (1980).

6. **Furstenberg, F.F.** *Unplanned parenthood: the social consequences of teenage childbearing.* New York, Free Press, 1979.
7. **Moore, K.A.** Teenage childbirth and welfare dependency. *Family planning perspectives,* **10**: 233–235 (1978).
8. **Rothman, D. & Capell, P.** Teenage pregnancy in England and Wales: some demographic and medico-social aspects. *Journal of biosocial science,* **10**(Suppl. 5): 65–83 (1978).
9. **O'Connell, M.** Comparative estimates of teenage illegitimacy in the United States, 1940–44 and 1970–74. *Demography,* **17**: 13–23 (1980).
10. **National Center for Health Statistics.** Teenage childbearing: United States 1966–75. *Monthly vital statistics reports,* **26**(Suppl.) (1977).
11. **Dunnell, K.** *Family formation, 1976.* London, H.M. Stationery Office, 1979.
12. **Ruzicka, L.T., ed.** *Nuptiality and fertility.* Liège, International Union for the Scientific Study of Population, 1982.
13. **Lewin, B.** Unmarried cohabitation: a marriage form in a changing society. *Journal of marriage and the family,* **44**: 763–773 (1982).
14. *Research needs and approaches in adolescent reproductive health in developing countries of the European Region:* report on a Working Group. Copenhagen, WHO Regional Office for Europe, 1980 (document ICP/MCH 023).
15. **Klasen, H.J. et al.** Oorzaken van brandwonden bij jonge kinderen. *Nederlands tijdschrift voor geneeskunde,* **122**: 1244–1248 (1978).
16. **Karwacki, J.J., Jr. & Baker, S.P.** Children in motor vehicles — never too young to die. *Journal of the American Medical Association,* **242**: 2848–2851 (1979).
17. **Richter, E.D.** Potential-years-life-lost from motor vehicle crashes in Israel: an epidemiological analysis. *International journal of epidemiology,* **8**: 383–388 (1979).
18. **Sjölin, S. & Smedby, B.** The state of health of Swedish children. *Acta paediatrica scandinavica,* **275**(Suppl.): 16–27 (1979).
19. **Meirik, O. et al.** Impact of changing age and parity distribution of mothers on perinatal mortality in Sweden, 1953–1975. *International journal of epidemiology,* **8**: 361–364 (1979).
20. **Holinger, P.C.** Violent deaths among the young: recent trends in suicide, homicide and accidents. *American journal of psychiatry,* **136**: 1144–1147 (1979).
21. **Mednick, S.A. & Christiansen, K.O., ed.** *Biosocial bases of criminal behaviour.* New York, Gardner Press, 1977.
22. **Olson, L.** Social and psychological correlates of pregnancy resolution among adolescent women: a review. *American journal of orthopsychiatry,* **50**: 432–445 (1980).
23. WHO Technical Report Series, No. 609, 1977 (*Health needs of adolescents*).
24. **Clausen, J.A. & Clausen, S.R.** The effects of family size on parents and children. *In*: Fawcett, J.T., ed. *Psychological perspectives on population.* New York, Basic Books Inc, 1973, pp. 185–208.

6

Implications of demographic change for the adult population (20–59 years)

S. Haberman & A.J. Fox

Changes over the past 50 years and in the next 20 years in marriage and divorce, in fertility, in mortality, in migration and in family living patterns will influence the circumstances and roles of adults in the year 2000. The purpose of this chapter is to discuss some of these influences; it is intended to provide the basis for discussion, not a definitive review.

Demographic changes among the young and the elderly alter the needs of these groups and hence their demands on the adult population. Demographic changes among those aged 20–59 years affect the ways in which they can respond to the immediate needs of the young and the elderly, and influence the demands that they are likely to make on their own children's generations when they themselves become old, as well as the quality of response of their children's generations when they reach adulthood. This feedback process will be referred to again later.

Circumstances and Roles of Adults

Fig. 1 is based on data obtained from the longitudinal study for England & Wales by the Office of Population Censuses and Surveys (*1*) (comprising a 1% sample taken from the 1971 census) and characterizes people according to "family status". Although cross-sectional, it indicates clearly the main transitions that take place between the ages of 15 and 60 years as individuals move through phases of the family life cycle. Most people start their young adult life still dependent on their parents. They establish their own homes either as newly married couples or alone but independent. At ages 30–49 years, over 60% of both sexes are in households comprising married couples with dependent children. A further 15–20% are married couples with no dependent children — either because they are childless or because their children have already left home. At ages 50–64 years the majority are married couples without dependent children (i.e. their children have now left home). The importance of alternative household structures becomes greater at older ages, especially for women, after the spouse has died. Some continue to live alone, but with increased age and progressive disability

Fig. 1. Distribution of people by usual place of residence and by family status

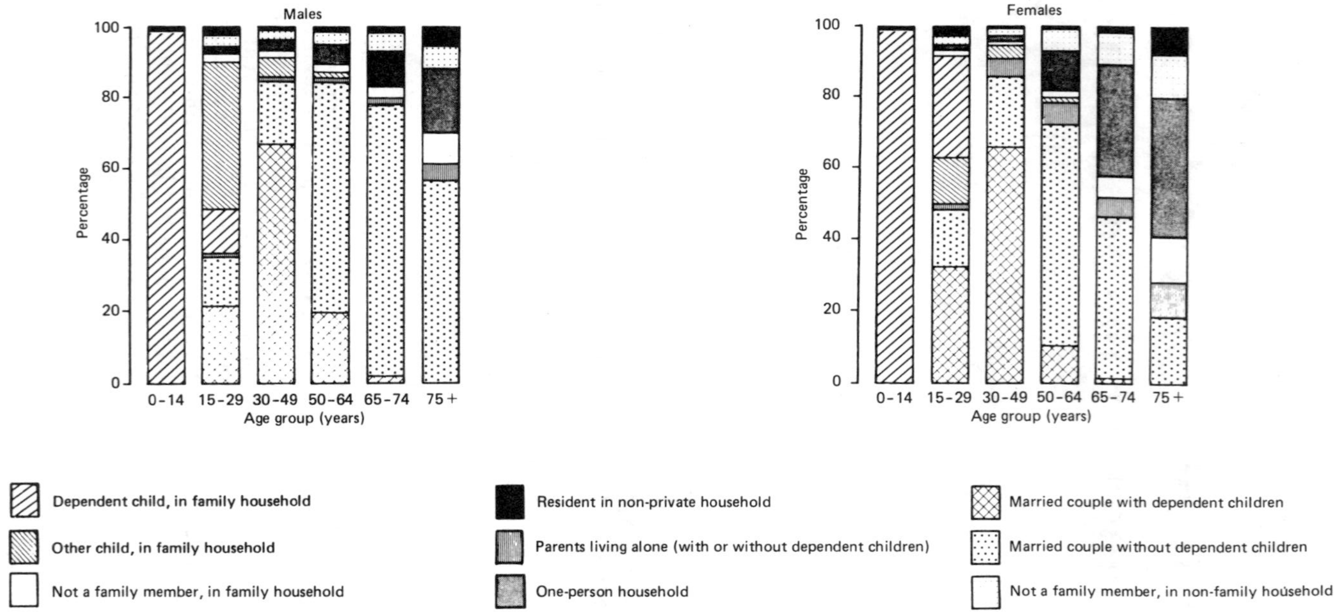

others will move to live with relatives or others, and an increasing proportion move into homes or hospitals. Thus Heikkinen, in Chapter 7 of this book, reports that about one quarter of those aged over 65 years live in one-person households, and about one quarter to one third live in joint households with a partner or children.

Using the basic model of the nuclear family life cycle (Table 1), changes over time in the structure of the family life cycle for several European countries can be examined (Fig. 2). Between 1950 and 1970, the life cycle lengthened because of the fall in mortality and the decrease in the average age at first marriage. Fig. 2 indicates that phase V is the longest, followed in general by phase III. The changes in the total length of the life cycle and the length of its different phases show that this increase leads to a relative increase in phases V and VI, with the relative increase in the former being the larger. Further, as completed family size decreases, so phases I/III and IV become shorter (and vice versa).

Table 1. Basic model of nuclear family life cycle

Phases of family life cycle	Events characterizing: beginning of phase	Events characterizing: end of phase
I Formation	Marriage	Birth of first child
II Extension	Birth of first child	Birth of last child
III Completed extension	Birth of last child	First child leaves parents' home
IV Contraction	First child leaves parents' home	Last child leaves parents' home
V Completed contraction	Last child leaves parents' home	First spouse dies
VI Dissolution	First spouse dies	Surviving spouse dies

Source: World Health Organization (*2*).

Parallel to this demographic life cycle, other life cycles can be identified: those that reflect personal requirements for schools and education (which peak at 5–15 years of age but do not necessarily fall to zero during adulthood); food (which peak at 15–20 years and are fairly level during adulthood); housing (which peak across the broad age group of 30–65 years); health services (which fall from a high level at birth to a minimum at about 20 years of age and which rise monotonically thereafter); and jobs (which show a broad peak across the ages 20–59 years).

The employed adult population supports the young, the old and the unemployed, not only in family and social terms but also in economic terms through social insurance schemes which provide child benefit, retirement pensions, and unemployment benefit.

Fig. 2. The length of the different phases of the family life cycle, 1950 and 1970

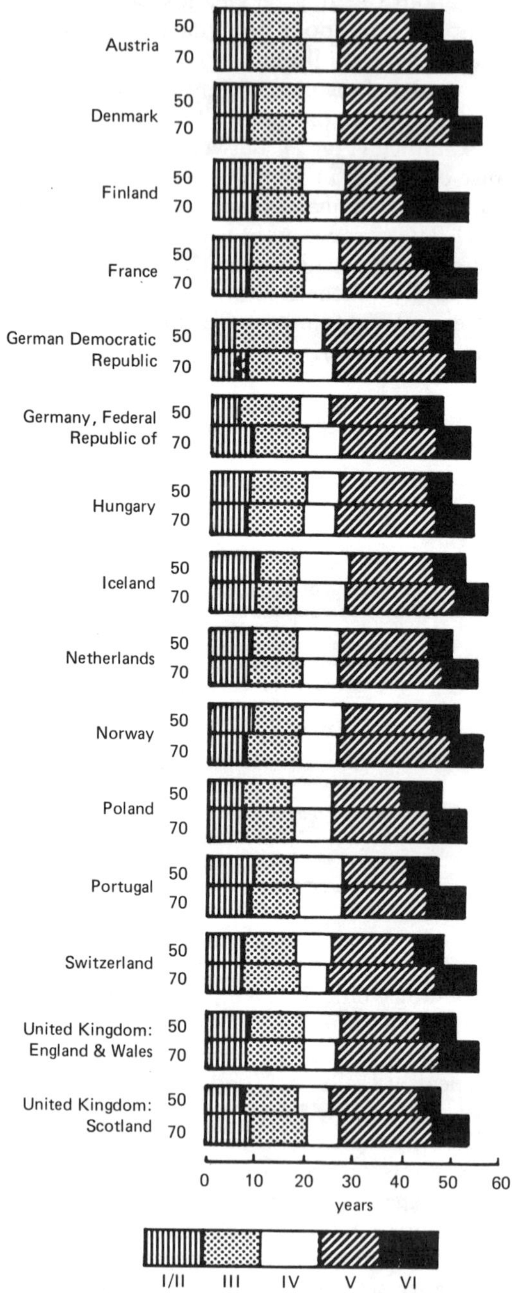

Source: World Health Organization (*2*).

During the last ten years the economic roles of adults have changed. For males, age-specific economic activity rates have remained steady (in the range 90–99%) with the rates, however, falling at 55–64 years of age, reflecting a trend towards earlier retirement. Owing to longer periods of formal education, the increased prevalence of single-parent families and of cohabitation, and the residual nature of the never-married group, non-married women have experienced a fall in economic activity. Married women show a rise at all ages, reflecting the increasing economic and social importance of the employment of married women, both part-time and full-time (*3*). Research indicates a high level of activity for married women before the birth of the first child and after the youngest child reaches the age of 10 or 11 years (*4*). Similarly, female participation in further and higher education has increased. The recent severe economic recession has produced very high levels of unemployment among young adults and removed many married women in marginal employment from the labour market, leading to a fall in activity rates.

The economy has been characterized by declining numbers employed in the manufacturing sector. This may be matched by a similar squeeze in the service sector, with high wages and improved technology encouraging employers to replace people with machines to raise productivity and profits. This description takes no account of the alternative economies (*5*) which simultaneously may gain in importance: the "black" economy, voluntary work, housework, household support, do-it-yourself, etc.

The housing circumstances of individuals are the major determinants of several aspects of the way people choose to live. First, they influence the ability of people to move, for example, in search of work or for support. Second, they affect people's willingness and ability to provide that support. Third, they determine the health of the young (e.g. through adventure playgrounds) and of the old (e.g. through heating and community centres).

Underlying many of the relationships within countries between the circumstances and experiences of specific groups will be socioeconomic and geographic differentials that reflect the importance of, for example, wealth, income and cultural background in determining these relationships.

Fertility

The number and timing of children in family units influences, among other things:

- the number of children dependent on young adults for support;
- the ages at which middle-aged adults no longer have responsibility for children (i.e. the start of phase V); and
- the amount of support available to help care for the elderly, mainly at ages after the children have left home.

The interrelation between fertility trends and the roles and circumstances of adults in the year 2000 will be discussed for three broad cohorts defined by their age range in that year.

Young adults (20–34 years)

Projections up to the year 2000 must be based on assumptions about the future childbearing experience of women currently aged under 20 years. Factors likely to influence their behaviour include their expectations and aspirations; changes in the economic climate; female employment patterns and prospects; participation of women (in particular) in higher education; reduced stillbirth and infant mortality rates; mortality rates for adolescents, in particular from road accidents; and the balance between the sexes and fluctuations in past birth rates, as this balance operates through the marriage market (it may also be affected by differential migration). These factors affect fertility through the voluntary practice of contraception — the ability of people to limit future fertility will be influenced by the continued availability of effective means of contraception and the development of new practices such as the increasing use of male sterilization.

Middle-aged adults (35–49 years)

For those at the younger end of this age group, many of the factors listed above will still be relevant. However, for many who will be in this age range in the year 2000, particularly those aged 45–49 years, their childbearing days will already be complete. Therefore the number and timing of their children are known and the proportions who will have reached particular ages by the year 2000 can be estimated.

The economic circumstances of these adults will to some extent be affected by their demographic experience. For example, the changes in fertility between 1960 and 1980 — involving a fall in completed family size and shorter intervals between births (*6*) — may have implications for the number of women entering the labour force, because they will no longer have the responsibility for children at home (even assuming no change in the attitude of married women to paid employment).

Older adults (50–59 years)

Fig. 1 suggests that older adults form the group on whom the initial needs of the elderly are liable to fall. The size of this group is determined by the childbearing experience of their parents (between 1935 and 1950). In England & Wales, changes in fertility between 1900 and 1935 and between 1935 and 1950 are characterized by a marked rise in the proportion of women who had two or more children; the proportion of zero- or one-child families for the 1912–1916 birth cohort of families was much higher than for the 1932–1936 birth cohort. This change is also reflected in a rise in the mean completed family size for birth cohorts (rising from 1.78 for those born in 1912–1916 to 2.19 for those born in 1932–1936). At the same time, for given family sizes there has been a tendency for babies to be born at younger maternal ages and closer together. These changes imply that there will be more children in this age group per elderly person, that these children will not have responsibility for their own children (who will have already left home) and that they will be closer in age to their parents. Therefore, assuming no change in attitudes towards parental support among people in this age group, parental support would be expected to increase.

Marriage, Divorce and Family Lifestyles

The principal medium through which adults provide support to older and younger generations is through family, household and kinship networks, e.g. people living under the same roof sharing resources, people living near to relatives or friends, children living with parents, and the elderly living with (adult) children.

Family formation occurs predominantly through marriage, although cohabitation has gained in popularity in many countries, particularly in Scandinavia. In England & Wales 10% of women aged 20–24 years who married in 1971–1975 cohabited before marriage, compared with only 1% of women of the same age group who married in 1956–1960 (*7*).

Family dissolution occurs principally through divorce or separation, with widowhood no longer important among those aged 20–59 years.

Prediction of family circumstances in the year 2000 will depend on future behaviour and not on direct extrapolations from the past. For young adults in the year 2000, how they choose to live (e.g. whether they cohabit, at which ages they decide to marry and their divorce rates) will influence the circumstances in which they bring up and support their children. For adults over 35 years of age in the year 2000, the magnitude and spread of their divorce and separation rates may be important factors in determining links with older generations (e.g. divorced women may return to live with their aged parents and provide the support supplied by spinsters to their parents in the early 1900s). In England & Wales the current high level of divorce is balanced by high remarriage rates, resulting in over 30% of divorcees remarrying within one year and 50% within four years (*8*). For adults aged over 35 in the year 2000, the extent of this remarriage will clearly be important, together with how remarriage rates move in sympathy with first marriage rates. By the turn of the century, alternative household structures may have become established to provide, for example for the elderly, independence and a limited degree of communal support when needed, or for the young a pooling of resources between more orthodox households for the communal support of children.

Mortality

The mortality of people aged 20–64 years has generally been falling. In particular, maternal mortality has virtually disappeared. At these ages, mortality can be associated with the social epidemics of smoking, motor transport accidents and suicide, which have already affected recent generations of males and are now beginning to affect females. The future trends should lead to a narrowing of the sex differential in mortality rates. For example, in England & Wales at ages 15–24 years, male mortality rates for accidents and violence fell by 3% between 1963 and 1979 but female rates rose by 27% (*9,10*).

The principal causes of death today are associated with a lower level of prior morbidity than formerly — thus, lung cancer, heart disease and accidents and violence are accompanied by shorter duration of prior morbidity than respiratory disease and tuberculosis. Mortality rates from these causes have either risen or fallen slowly over the last 20 years (*11*).

Mortality among those aged 20–64 years can therefore be expected to have a lower impact on this age group and its ability to support the dependent and needy in other age groups. But reductions in mortality at these ages for people who will be elderly in the year 2000 will contribute to an increased burden for subsequent generations.

The steep decline in infant mortality and stillbirth rates, and also the improved screening of births for congenital malformations, should lead to more children surviving infancy and childhood in a healthier condition, thus reducing the burden on their parents (e.g. the prevalence of Down's syndrome should be reduced).

The trends in mortality in those under 20 years have an effect on the sex ratio of the numbers surviving to adulthood. Thus, the tendency towards a balance between the sexes, followed by an excess of unmarried young adults will have repercussions for future marriage and fertility.

Migration

The effects of international migration on European countries need to be discussed in terms of both the importing and exporting country. The first generation of such migrants comprise young adults, possibly males initially, and families including children. In the receiving country, the early problems of fitting in to the new society will usually involve the formation of geographical clusters of communities, probably within the inner cities. As time goes on, immigrants tend to adopt the childbearing, morbidity and mortality patterns of the native population. This partly reflects selection among the migrants and partly changes in their expectations and aspirations. Immigration may correct a deficiency in the age/sex structure of the native population in the receiving country. Thus, the arrival of young adult males into a country with a prior excess of single adult women would enable more single women to marry (for example, the experience of Belgium and France after the Second World War). For the children of immigrants, the problems are primarily concerned with education in schools and poor housing. Later assimilation may lead to a change in geographic dispersion and levels of childbearing similar to those of the native population. At this stage, some emigration to the country of origin may take place. Ultimately, aged dependants may follow, to be supported in the new country or be supported financially at a distance by remittances sent home. The same is true of wives and children at the early stage of the process.

Much of this type of migration in recent years has been related to work opportunities in the richer countries and involved movements from, for example, Greece, Ireland, Morocco, Portugal, Spain, Turkey and the New Commonwealth to Belgium, France, the Federal Republic of Germany, the Netherlands, Scandinavia, Switzerland and the United Kingdom. The immediate effect on the country of destination is to provide cheap labour and facilitate economic progress. The long-term effects associated with the problems of social integration of succeeding generations have yet to be seen.

Alternatively, the effect on the country of origin is to remove a considerable fraction of its productive manpower and possibly ease temporarily unemployment problems and provide some economic benefit from remittances sent back home. But these benefits are again short-term. Some countries, such as Ireland, have traditionally exported large numbers of people and hence been able to enjoy high fertility rates without rapid population growth.

Internal migration may be seen in terms of the timing within the family life cycle — leaving the parental home, having children, seeking employment, retiring, support for the elderly. Internal migration has important effects on ties between generations, in particular the provision of family support for the elderly, young adults moving away from the parental home to seek employment or participate in further/higher education, the migration of newly retired married couples, and their return on bereavement or when in need.

Economic changes and development also affect internal migration through the search for work. Much of this flow is projected to occur from rural to urban areas.

General Policy Issues

Employment

Present economic projections indicate that European countries will require considerably smaller workforces in the generation of material wealth, which will itself derive less from steel construction and shipbuilding and other central industries and more from light, high technology industries such as electronics. This will have serious implications, including a reduced period of life spent at work, shorter working hours, increased leisure and pressure to restrict employment opportunities for women. Greater occupational mobility will be essential, and this may require major retraining programmes and participation of mature students in higher education on a part-time as well as full-time basis. The unskilled may create special problems as they fall further behind in a society that is becoming increasingly technological.

Mention has been made of the growth of alternative economies based on housework and skills acquired at home or at leisure. This could be fostered by the increased availability of labour and, *inter alia*, the increased "need" created by the numbers of elderly with their special problems and impairments. They may well receive greater recognition, and incentive schemes could be developed for them.

The importance of higher economic participation for women has been mentioned. If this participation is to continue at a high level, if not increase further, then greater flexibility in working conditions will be required to allow married couples greater freedom in deciding on their respective roles and the timing of their participation in the labour force.

The changes in employment patterns will continue to affect the social structure as societies become more white collar and less blue collar dominated. This again has wide implications for behaviour and the circumstances of adults in the year 2000, particularly when these are determined by social background and attitudes.

These changes will vary from country to country, each of which will determine its own responses, reflecting partly its past demographic trends and population structure and partly its social, economic and cultural structure.

Housing

One of the major determinants of the choice people make in terms of their lifestyle, including family structure, is their housing circumstances. Forward projections of housing (by type and geographic location) may be used to indicate stresses that are likely to be encountered and will identify the need for initiatives — for example, if alternative methods of supporting the elderly are to be sought. Shortages of housing could have implications for the first marriage rates of young couples, or result in couples marrying but living with parents.

Possible changes in tenancy practice could also have important implications. For example, the rise in owner-occupation and council housing at the expense of private rented accommodation could particularly affect the attractiveness or otherwise of family support for the elderly. Also, tax changes may have important effects; for example, the gradual erosion in England & Wales in the real value of the maximum amount of mortgage interest qualifying for income tax relief may alter the pattern of tenure. Furthermore, it may affect the economy directly, since capital may be freed from being tied up in the family home for investment as equity capital to support new industries, etc.

Low fertility

Low fertility over the past 20 years and the possibility of its continuation during the next two decades has implications for the numbers of children dependent on the adult population, and for the ultimate size of the adult population that will be required to support increasing numbers of the very old (i.e. those over 85 years of age).

After the year 2000, the adult population will be required to support fewer children but an increasing number of the elderly. With time, the dependency ratio may be expected to fall and then rise monotonically as the cohort effect passes through. One aspect of dependency is support through social insurance, with the employed population being taxed to pay pensions, unemployment benefit and child benefit. The amount of this tax could rise dramatically as the workforce contracts for economic and demographic reasons while the quantity spent on pensions (especially if the retirement age falls) and unemployment benefit rises (*12,13*).

Divorce

Divorce rates are currently at unprecedentedly high levels, with about 20% of marriages ultimately ending in divorce. The likely continuation of these high rates could present problems relating to single-parent families which in time could affect, *inter alia*, the social integration of children. This could also emphasize the need for more flexible housing patterns to minimize hardship and disruption following family break-up.

Mortality and morbidity

Wider sex differentials among those currently aged 20–59 years may lead to a change in the future supply of and demand for support, affecting both the social and the health services. Given the nature of the principal causes of death in this age group, the role of preventive health education is likely to increase (e.g. the wearing of safety helmets and car seat belts, anti-smoking campaigns, improved nutrition, and increased but moderate physical activity).

Mobility

Linked to economic change is the probable regional development of those poorer areas within the European countries. This is likely to have an impact on the direction and intensity of migrational flow and lead to changes in the socioeconomic and demographic differentials that exist between regions. The estimated trend towards increasing urbanization will have serious implications for the social structure within conurbations, the decay currently occurring in the nuclei of these areas, and the current growth taking place on the peripheries of cities.

References

1. **Fox, A.J. & Goldblatt, P.O.** *Longitudinal study 1971–1975: socio-demographic mortality differentials.* London, H.M. Stationery Office, 1982 (OPCS LS No. 1).
2. *Health and the family: studies on the demography of family life cycles and their health implications.* Geneva, World Health Organization, 1978.
3. Labour force outlook to 1986. *Department of Employment gazette,* **89**: 167–173 (1981).
4. **Joshi, H. & Owen, S.** *Demographic predictors of women's work participation in post-war Britain.* London, London School of Hygiene and Tropical Medicine, 1981 (Centre for Population Studies Working Paper No. 81).
5. **Gershuny, J.I. & Pahl, R.E.** Britain in the decade of the three economies. *New society,* 3 Jan. 1980, pp. 7–9.
6. **Britton, M.** Birth intervals. *Population trends,* **18**: 8–16 (1979).
7. **Dunnell, K.** *Family formation, 1976.* London, H.M. Stationery Office, 1979.
8. **Leete, R. & Anthony, S.** Divorce and remarriage: a record linkage study. *Population trends,* **16**: 5–11 (1979).
9. *Statistical review for England and Wales for 1963. Part 1, medical.* London, H.M. Stationery Office, 1965.
10. *Mortality statistics: cause, 1979.* London, H.M. Stationery Office, 1980 (Series DH2 No. 6).
11. *Trends in mortality 1951–75.* London, H.M. Stationery Office, 1978 (Series DH1 No. 3).
12. **Ermisch, J.** Paying the piper: demographic changes and pension contributions. *Policy studies,* **1**: 213–220 (1981).
13. **Hemming, R. & Kay, J.A.** The cost of the state earnings related pension scheme. *Economic journal,* **92**: 300–319 (1982).

7

Implications of demographic change for the elderly population (60 years and over)

E. Heikkinen

The purpose of this chapter is to examine, in the light of the main demographic trends, the status and prospects of old people in various European countries. Some developmental trends in the status of the elderly appear to be rather similar in most of these countries. Urbanization, industrialization, development of production, differentiation between occupations and other well known changes have created social and cultural conditions that influence the way of life of the elderly in much the same manner. Included among these changes are the development of pension systems and comprehensive welfare services, the trend towards smaller families, increasing social mobility, and growing demand for new cultural and leisure activities.

On the other hand, the European countries are at different stages of industrialization and urbanization. The proportion of the population aged 65 years and over varies from about 10% to about 14% between different geographic areas (Table 1) and in some countries the proportion is as high as 17%. The percentage of rural dwellers aged 70 years and over among the total population varies greatly among the different regions of Europe (Table 2). Elderly people are commonly overrepresented in rural areas in highly industrialized countries. According to the available predictions, the proportion of the urban population will increase by about 10% between 1975 and the year 2000, the change being greatest in Southern and Eastern Europe.

Variations in cultural traditions have a marked influence on the living conditions of the elderly. The development of public services and other forms of social policy is claimed to weaken traditional primary structures. This is seen to arise, for example, as changes in the function of the family in the context of systems of care, according to the developmental state of a given country (*3*).

In addition, the social, political and economic restructuring that has occurred in the socialist countries has greatly affected all societal institutions and thus also the living conditions of old people. Provisions for the health care and wellbeing of the elderly are incorporated into the constitutions of the socialist countries of Eastern Europe. Also, different geographical circumstances can influence the solutions that are adopted for the care of the elderly.

Table 1. Percentages of people aged 65 and over in Europe: the situation in 1975 and projections to the year 2000

Region	Year		
	1975	1985	2000
Europe, total	12.1	12.3	14.2
Eastern Europe (except the USSR)	11.4	10.8	13.2
Northern Europe	13.7	14.7	14.6
Southern Europe	10.4	11.2	14.2
Western Europe	13.6	13.3	14.9
USSR	8.9	9.6	12.0

Source: Bourgeois-Pichat, J. (*1*).

A major problem in exploring how old people live is the scantiness of cross-national studies, and the consequent difficulties in undertaking comparative analyses on the effects of demographic change on the living conditions of the aged. Only a broad indication of various developmental trends can therefore be presented. Furthermore, their interpretation is rendered difficult by substantial variations in ideology, by the historical and social state of development of a given country, and by differences in the organizational approaches used to meet the needs and demands of old people.

Changing Patterns of Needs and Interests

The situation of the elderly in the industrialized countries is continuously changing in relation to the economic and cultural development of those societies. Marked differences exist in various aspects of life between generations. People born at the beginning of the century have witnessed considerable economic and social progress which has reduced poverty and in many other ways improved living conditions. These people, when interviewed, commonly express substantial satisfaction with life.

One positive consequence of the changing age structure has been an increase in the research effort devoted to the solution of the problems of the aged. Several aspects of the situation of the elderly have been investigated in most of the European countries. The most common questions that have been analysed deal with housing conditions, income maintenance, social integration, health status, need for services, and overall satisfaction with life. On the basis of such research, it has been possible to identify "risk groups" which have then received greater attention from the various service systems.

Housing

The housing situation of the elderly encompasses such aspects as the standard of housing, characteristics of household composition, and the effects of the neighbourhood and the environment on the wellbeing of the elderly (*4–7*).

Table 2. Percentages of the rural and urban populations aged 70 years and over by major European region, 1975 and 2000

Population	Europe, total			Eastern Europe			Northern Europe			Southern Europe			Western Europe		
	1975	2000	Change	1975	2000	Change	1975	2000	Change	1975	2000	Change	1975	2000	Change
Rural	2.41	2.00	-0.41	3.18	2.87	- 0.31	1.45	0.99	-0.46	2.68	2.31	- 0.37	2.07	1.50	-0.57
Urban															
Men	63.1	72.2	+9.1	51.0	62.3	+11.8	78.9	85.1	+6.2	49.9	64.1	+14.2	72.9	80.6	+7.7
Women	69.6	78.3	+8.7	56.8	68.3	+12.0	85.6	91.6	+6.0	55.5	69.2	+13.7	78.2	86.3	+8.1

Source: United Nations (*2*).

Most elderly persons (80–90%) live independently in their own households. In Sweden, for example, about 90% of people aged 65 and over live in ordinary apartments, and in Finland about 85% live in ordinary houses. Among the older age groups, the proportion living in institutions or in houses specifically constructed for the elderly is markedly higher: in Sweden about 60% of those aged 85–89 years live in their own households.

Whilst the standard of housing of old people has improved considerably, it is still lower than that enjoyed by younger generations. This situation partly reflects cohort differences: new independent generations generally begin with a higher standard of housing than the previous generation. A standard of housing that is below average is particularly evident in rural areas and in the central areas of larger cities. There are, however, exceptions such as Greece, where the major housing problems are found in big cities; in rural areas on the contrary, it has been reported that there are no acute housing problems for old people (*8*).

Data about housing preferences support the commonly held view that old people want to live in their own homes, in a familiar neighbourhood, and in close contact with their relatives and friends. On the other hand the younger generations, who were born into and have lived in welfare states, seem to perceive many problems in the organization and quality of their lives.

The members of every new generation perceive their lives through their own experience and in the framework of the situation in which they are living. Differences between the needs and interests of the cohorts are great. Also, within any one cohort social disparity tends to increase with advancing age. In this context it should be remembered that variations in state of health, social integration, maintenance of income, need for services, etc. that are observed between different people in old age are not causally related to old age itself, but rather are the end result of an individual's entire lifespan.

Retirement is reported to accentuate these differences and emphasize the difficulties of groups who are especially disadvantaged, the ill-protected, the small farmers and agricultural workers, the small firms in industry and commerce, and people in service occupations, who obtained compensation allowances only very late in life. The position of women, and particularly of very old women, is even worse (*3*). Each new generation that attains retirement age can be expected to be better educated, healthier and functionally more capable of performing various activities than the previous ones. On the other hand some data suggest that differences in the prevalence of certain common diseases between various social classes have not diminished during recent decades, even though the general health of the populations under investigation may have improved (*9*). These and other similar observations emphasize the need to direct societal measures towards the prevention of ill health and social deprivation long before old age is attained, in addition to measures specifically developed for the care of the elderly.

The changes that have occurred in most of the European countries have increased the number of one-person households (particularly among elderly women), lengthened the distances between parents and children, and forced the elderly to move to new environments. These processes will continue in the future, with likely harmful effects on the elderly, if new societal measures to counter them are not developed. It has been estimated that about one quarter of those over 65 in several Western European countries live in one-person households (*3*). In Eastern European countries 9–17% of people aged 60 and over live alone (*4*).

The family today still plays an important role in the social relationships of the elderly. In some European countries, such as Poland, nearly 70% of people aged 65 and over who have children live with them. In other socialist countries, especially Bulgaria, Romania and the USSR (particularly in the republics of the Caucasus and Middle Asia), extended families are still common (*10*). In the more industrialized countries the figures are lower: about 40% in Great Britain and 20% in Denmark, for example (*11*). In the European part of the USSR the proportion of extended families is only 10–20%. In Poland, even outside the agricultural areas, the proportion of old people living with children is more than 50%, and older people are more willing to live with children than is the case in many Western European countries. Furthermore, the proportion of the elderly in Poland living with a relative at the beginning of the 1970s was 76% among peasants, 58% among workers and 55% among employees (*12*). In the Netherlands, less than 2% of the aged wish to live with their children (*13*). In many societies, the elderly prefer to maintain separate households from their relatives, but at the same time would like their relatives to live close enough to permit regular contact — in other words "intimacy at a distance".

Most countries have developed measures and service systems to improve the housing conditions of the elderly in order to increase their independence and to prevent premature institutionalization. These include renovation programmes for old houses, sheltered dwellings and a range of auxiliary support measures. It is now widely recognized that appropriate housing conditions and the quality of the environment have greater importance for continuity of life among the elderly compared with younger people. In fact, many problems of the elderly could be dealt with by improving their standard of housing and ensuring access to service systems. In countries such as Sweden, where intensive programmes have been developed to improve the housing conditions of the elderly, 90% of them can live in ordinary dwellings despite the fact that the proportion of people aged 65 and over is one of the highest in Europe.

Social integration and mode of life

The social networks and cultural activities of the elderly have undergone marked changes during recent decades. A new social role of pensioner has developed, and on a macrosocial level the formation of a subculture of the elderly can be seen with their own clubs, associations and political organizations. Some features of this restructuring of the social networks of the elderly may be antagonistic towards the rest of society if the elderly feel that their justified demands are not met.

About one quarter to one third of old people feel loneliness and anomie, and are socially isolated or have too little communication and contacts. The majority of the elderly can, however, maintain social activities and interests at the same level as before (*14,15*). With advancing age official social participation and activities outside the home seem to decrease, and unofficial social participation and activities at home appear to increase. The elderly who belong to the higher social classes and are more educated are more involved in social activities and cultural interests than others.

Adaptation to, and training for, retirement are among the most important issues in social gerontology. In an international comparative study concentrating on the lifestyles of retired teachers in seven countries, and steel industry workers in four countries, it was observed that post-retirement life continued very much in the same vein as before but with a slower tempo (*16*). Clearly, there is an increasing need to prepare elderly workers for retirement, and specific programmes have been developed for this purpose in different countries. The aim of preparation for retirement is to raise the level of adaptation to a new period of life and thus prevent medical and social problems.

The average life expectancy at the age of 65 is already as long as childhood, and this period will presumably become even longer if the current decline in mortality among the elderly continues and if the retirement age is lowered. Educational programmes are also needed for retired people to prevent social isolation and to stimulate them to participate in various spheres of social life.

Very little is known about the content of, and changes in, the mode of life of retired people. The studies carried out so far have usually focused on specific aspects such as satisfaction with life and living habits. It has been shown that general satisfaction with life is correlated with social participation, socioeconomic conditions, and level of health (*15,17–19*).

Age differences in the propensity for various living habits have been analysed in several studies. These have shown, among other findings, that physical activity tends to decrease with advancing age and also that the prevalence of smoking is lower among the elderly compared with younger people (*12,20,21*). Possible changes in living habits during the historical development of the societies under study have not been investigated, and cross-national studies are totally lacking. Some observations suggest that even old people are able to modify their behaviour if cultural developments, such as for example new health education programmes, encourage behavioural changes. This can be seen in the increased interest in physical training among the elderly in the industrialized welfare states such as the Nordic countries and the Federal Republic of Germany.

Solidarity among family members still seems to be high and the family has retained the major part of its economic, protective and emotional functions. About 80% of the elderly in several European countries have children living no more than half an hour's walking or driving distance away. Data of this kind do not, however, reveal anything about the quality of family relations, which presumably have changed together with the functions of the family. Some research findings suggest that the development of special services for the elderly (about 30 different service categories in several countries) may lead to a situation in which children are less interested in helping their parents. In Finland, a growing number of old people seem to prefer assistance from the official services instead of receiving help from their children. How future social policy can maintain a proper balance between the resources of the professional services and resources of the family is a question that has important implications for family relations.

Health and functional ability

The development of the health status of the elderly is not well known. As Table 3 illustrates, the increase in life expectancy at age 65 has been a gradual process and is at present more than 15 years for women and more than 13 years for men in several European countries. Mortality is also declining among the aged in many countries (see Table 4) and some recent findings suggest that, particularly during the last few years, the decline has been quite rapid, particularly among women (*23–25*).

Table 3. Mean life expectancy at age 65 at the beginning of the century and in the 1970s in selected European countries

Country	Period	Men		Women	
		Mean life expectancy	Increase	Mean life expectancy	Increase
Belgium	1891-1900	10.6		11.6	
	1968-1972	12.1	1.5	15.3	3.7
Denmark	1901-1905	11.9		13.0	
	1977-1978	13.9	2.0	17.6	4.6
Finland	1901-1910	10.8		11.9	
	1978	12.3	1.5	16.3	4.4
France	1898-1903	13.3		14.6	
	1977	13.7	0.4	17.9	3.3
Germany	1901-1910	10.4		11.1	
German Democratic Republic	1976	12.2	1.8	14.8	3.7
Germany, Federal Republic of	1976-1978	12.6	2.2	16.2	5.1
Iceland	1901-1910	11.7		13.4	
	1977-1978	16.2	4.5	18.9	5.5
Italy	1901-1911	10.7		10.8	
	1970-1972	13.3	2.6	16.2	5.4
Netherlands	1900-1909	11.6		12.3	
	1977	13.9	2.3	18.0	5.7
Norway	1901-1910	13.5		14.4	
	1977-1978	14.3	0.8	17.7	3.3
Scotland	1891-1900	10.5		11.5	
	1971-1973	11.9	1.4	15.2	3.7
Sweden	1901-1910	12.8		13.7	
	1978	14.2	1.4	17.7	4.0

Source: Central Statistical Office of Finland (*22*).

Table 4. Age-specific mortality per 1000 population during the 1930s and 1970s in selected European countries

Country	Period	Sex	Age group					
			60-64	65-69	70-74	75-79	80-84	85+
England & Wales	1930-1932	M	29.2	46.5	74.4		149.9	
		F	21.4	33.8	55.5		128.7	
	1976	M	24.9	40.3	65.1	100.7	153.5	249.9
		F	12.6	19.8	33.7	58.1	103.8	201.4
Finland	1930-1932	M	34.1	47.0	67.4	95.6	125.5	159.5
		F	22.4	33.3	56.3	89.8	135.7	189.0
	1977	M	29.0	43.4	64.1	96.0	149.3	222.3
		F	11.0	18.0	32.4	59.2	99.1	190.6
France	1930-1932	M	33.0	50.1		123.0		
		F	21.6	35.4		103.0		
	1976	M	20.4	34.0	53.9	89.2	140.3	251.3
		F	8.1	14.4	25.5	49.3	91.5	202.0
Germany	1937	M	26.7	41.8		102.2		
		F	21.6	36.0		97.1		
German Democratic Republic	1976	M	23.8	39.8	66.3	105.3	161.4	283.6
		F	12.6	22.4	41.2	73.5	129.6	248.9
Germany, Federal Republic of	1977	M	23.0	37.6	61.8	94.4	142.8	228.6
		F	10.9	17.9	32.5	58.8	104.7	196.5
Hungary	1930-1932	M	30.0	46.3	74.1		160.2	
		F	25.3	41.9	66.8		150.8	
	1977	M	26.7	42.1	68.5	107.0	161.3	251.9
		F	14.4	24.3	41.8	73.7	123.2	219.6
Iceland	1940	M	19.3	32.1	54.2		121.8	
		F	12.5	24.0	41.0		112.7	
	1977	M	14.2	22.0	42.2	57.3	95.9	169.2
		F	6.1	13.2	26.4	33.8	83.2	141.0
Italy	1930-1932	M	26.1	40.7	67.3		145.2	
		F	21.4	35.3	59.6		135.5	
	1976	M	21.4	34.5	54.7	88.7	135.7	232.5
		F	10.0	17.1	30.0	58.7	107.9	199.1
Netherlands	1930-1932	M	22.2	36.1	59.1		131.4	
		F	21.0	33.6	56.4		126.5	
	1977	M	20.2	33.6	52.4	78.1	116.1	194.3
		F	8.9	14.8	25.5	46.8	80.3	164.4
Poland	1933-1934	M	35.5	57.5	76.4		145.5	
		F	27.2	40.4	66.8		134.5	
	1977	M	26.0	40.3	63.3	95.5	144.4	203.9
		F	12.4	20.2	35.7	62.7	109.1	174.9
Portugal	1930-1932	M	29.7	45.9	74.0		155.6	
		F	20.1	32.3	56.6		140.8	
	1975	M	24.5	37.6	58.5	101.2	178.3	338.4
		F	11.2	19.6	35.2	72.2	138.2	259.1
Sweden	1930-1932	M	21.9	34.3	53.5	81.1	147.4	253.0
		F	18.9	30.5	50.3	58.7	100.0	182.8
	1976	M	18.2	30.0	50.0	80.8	128.3	230.8
		F	9.2	14.8	27.2	50.6	91.7	187.6
Switzerland	1930-1932	M	33.2	50.9	76.2		154.8	
		F	23.8	39.6	65.0		141.8	
	1977	M	17.9	31.6	47.9	77.3	122.3	212.6
		F	8.1	13.8	24.9	47.2	84.7	177.1

Source: Central Statistical Office of Finland (*22*).

An overview of the state of health of the elderly depends, of course, on the method of examination. In careful clinical examination, an average of about nine diseases per person was found in a group of elderly patients (*26*). On the other hand, the average number of diseases that require medical treatment in a population aged 65 and over is about 2.5 per person (*27*). Surveys have commonly found that the prevalence of certain diseases (e.g. heart insufficiency) is higher than that observed in clinical examinations, and some other diseases can be diagnosed only through clinical examination (*28–30*). Chronic conditions comprise the majority of the diseases of the elderly. Moreover, the elderly would appear to change their aspirations about health and accept some symptoms and degenerative states as part of the normal process of aging, since only 30–40% of old people feel that they are healthy (*31–32*).

The assessment of the functional abilities of the elderly is important in order to provide them with adequate services and rehabilitative measures. Low functional status is particularly a problem among very old women and, because their number is constantly increasing, this problem will require more attention in the future from the point of view both of research and of social practice.

The state of health of the elderly and their perception of health may be assumed to vary between different cultures and in relation to the level of service systems. However, it is not possible to generalize further on the basis of the present research data. According to an interview study in Yugoslavia, about 70% of a group of urban people aged 60 years and over had three or more chronic diseases. In one town in the USSR, about 54% of those aged 60–64 years had three or more chronic conditions, and in the age group 75–79 years the corresponding figure, based on medical examination, was 92% (*12*).

Health and social services

In recent years there has been a rapid development of services in most European countries aimed at meeting the needs of the growing numbers of old people (*33*). In several countries the proportion of resources allocated to the health care of the elderly is more than 50% of all health care expenditure. The use of services among the aged is 3–4 times that expected on the basis of their proportion of the population. This situation has raised several important questions. How will the health status of the elderly develop in the future? What can be done to prevent premature disability and institutionalization? How should resources be divided among the different forms of health and social services, among families and among the elderly themselves? What factors can predict the development of the health and wellbeing of the elderly? Research into these questions is under way in many countries and policies for the aged are being planned and implemented to meet their most acute needs.

The main principle in the development of services is integration; that is, services intended for all members of society should also satisfy the needs of the elderly. The actual development of services has, however, led to an increasing number of services specifically planned for old people (*3,34,35*).

The rationale for this development lies in the processes of aging, which create new and complex demands on service systems, and also in the rapid changes in the environment that require the elderly to adapt beyond their capability to do so without outside assistance. The result has been a tendency towards a more and more marked differentiation and compartmentalization of the range of services offered (*3*). Various attempts have been made to systematize services in order to be able to respond as effectively as possible to the living conditions of the elderly (*36,37*).

One model for the systematization of services is built upon changes in roles with aging, on the needs of the elderly, and on the liberation of old people's own mental and physical resources. Four different categories of service emerge from the analysis.

- Services preserving the continuity of lifestyle. These are services catering for basic vital needs such as housing, health, information and work opportunities.

- Compensating services, which help the elderly in coping with the activities of daily life and in communicating with the outside world.

- Life-enhancing services, which try to satisfy needs of a higher order and aim to motivate a search for the new (opportunity creating services).

- Care services when health and functional abilities are lost.

This model implies a necessity to develop service systems by interlocking various forms of service to a flexible totality that can respond to the unique needs of every individual. People are generally old after they reach 75 years, when the processes of aging start to manifest themselves in various bodily tissues and functions. Before attaining that age an individual may incur disability, but this is mainly due to symptoms caused by a variety of diseases which in principle do not belong to normal aging. On reaching the age of 75 years there is a progressive development of general impairment, loss of working capacity and in some cases loss of ability for self-help (*10*). The need for periodic or continuous outside assistance for the elderly is steadily growing.

Recent demographic data indicate that in several countries the proportion of people aged 60–74 years is stagnating, whereas the proportion of old people (≧75 years) is rapidly increasing. The proportion of people aged 80 and over among those aged 60 and over is expected to increase from 10% to 14% between 1960 and the year 2000 (Table 5). The state of health of those aged 60–74 years is expected to improve in the future, and the main target for services will be those of a higher age, particularly women, who often have multiple morbidity and serious limitations in functional abilities.

Service systems in the future will also have to deal with problems of social disparity among the elderly. Education, previous professional status, place of residence, household composition and family relations, level of income, etc. influence the wellbeing of old people in a complex manner.

Table 5. Percentages of people aged over 80 years among those aged over 60 years, 1960 to 2000

Region	Year				
	1960	1970	1980	1990	2000
Europe, total	9.9	10.6	12.5	14.5	13.4
Eastern Europe (except the USSR)	8.2	8.6	11.2	13.3	11.2
Northern Europe	11.2	11.7	12.7	15.1	16.5
Southern Europe	9.7	10.9	11.5	13.4	13.1
Western Europe	10.3	11.1	14.1	16.1	13.5
USSR	9.6	10.1	11.9	14.0	12.7

Source: United Nations (*2*).

There also seem to be class-specific differences in perception of, access to, and use of services (*3*).

Medical, social and psychological factors combine in a series of reciprocal relationships to determine the development of the health and functional abilities of the elderly. Any system of services will probably fail if it is not able to perceive an old person as a totality comprising all the above-mentioned dimensions. The service system has also to achieve a balance between the privacy of old people and the active provision of services to those who objectively are in need of them but, for various reasons, do not use them.

An Aging Population: A Burden or a Resource?

An aging population would scarcely matter from the economic and social point of view, if the behaviour or attitudes of the members of the population were not closely linked with age (*38*). Past and future demographic trends suggest that most European countries are almost stationary as regards generation replacement. Many countries are moving towards a very low level of mortality and, in particular, there has been a sharp decline in mortality among the very old (*39*). The dependency ratio (the proportion of people aged 0–14 years plus the proportion of people aged 60 years and over to the population aged 15–59 years) will still decrease slightly in many countries during the last decades of this century because the increase in the proportion of the elderly has not yet offset the fall in the proportion of young people (Table 6). It can be assumed that this drop in the dependency ratio will make it possible to increase productivity, provided that available resources are effectively utilized. The situation may, however, change when the large generations born after the war reach retirement age.

Table 6. Dependency ratios in different regions of Europe, 1960 to 2000

Region	Year				
	1960	1970	1980	1990	2000
Europe, total	67.3	71.1	64.4	63.4	66.9
Eastern Europe (except the USSR)	68.6	67.4	63.0	66.1	65.0
Northern Europe	68.1	73.7	69.1	64.4	66.2
Southern Europe	65.2	54.8	65.4	65.2	48.8
Western Europe	67.8	74.0	62.1	59.2	66.8
USSR	68.8	68.3	59.7	67.5	70.2

Source: United Nations (*2*).

The current high level of unemployment in several Western European countries may cause increased tension between the economically active and the older population groups. The older labour force is criticized for its lack of mobility, rigidity and the outdated nature of its education. Gerontological research has shown that the processes of aging do not automatically lead to a decline in performance in all physiological functions, and that in several psychological and social tasks older workers, by means of experience and watchfulness, manage better than younger ones (*40*).

Predictions concerning the participation of persons aged 65 and over in the labour force suggest that the proportion of economically active men in this age group will fall from about 25% at present to about 12% by the year 2000. In many countries, e.g. Finland, the proportion of economically active people over 65 years of age is at present only about 5%. Opposite trends have also been reported, as for example in the USSR where the level of pensioners' employment has increased over the past decade while attempts have been made to facilitate the working conditions of older people (*32*). Large regional differences are also evident in the USSR in the proportion of workers who are active in production during the first pensionable 5-year period. These range from 50–60% in the Baltic republics to 15–20% in the republics of Middle Asia.

In future, the industrialized and urbanized societies will increasingly face the problem of how to maintain meaningful social roles for the elderly and how to create services to help old people not only to cope with the activities of daily life, but also to enable them to use their personal mental and physical resources for their own self-development and, in consequence, for the benefit of society at large. These questions were emphasized at the World Assembly on Aging held in Vienna in 1982 (*41*). The success of this task will depend on social, economic and cultural developments in the different societies. In some countries, even the provision of basic material security for the elderly is problematic, while in others the problems centre more on the spiritual needs of the aged.

In conclusion, a number of critical, perhaps even provocative statements about factors thought to be crucial in determining the development of health and mode of life among old people are listed below.

1. European societies are not suficiently prepared to face and handle the challenges brought about by the aging of their populations.

2. Views on the past conditions of the elderly tend to be romantic and over-optimistic. In several countries the prevalence of extended families has not been as common as is usually assumed, and even where it is common there are often serious psychosocial problems. On the other hand, the problems of the elderly are either overemphasized or their capacities and possibilities are regarded with an unrealistic optimism.

3. Gerontological research and training programmes should be strengthened. Current research does not meet the need for new knowledge about the processes of aging and the importance of the problems of the aged. In medicine, for example, the allocation of resources to gerontological research is minimal, even though the elderly are the main consumers of medical services. Training in gerontology and geriatrics is insufficient to provide medical and social workers with adequate knowledge, a positive attitude and proper skills to serve old people and to develop appropriate service systems. With regard to the processes of aging and the situation of the elderly, the principle of evolution should be adapted to research and training.

4. The condition of the elderly is a complex question which is inextricably intertwined with all spheres of social life. Therefore a long-term policy should be tailored to each society, comprising the physical, psychological and social dimensions of the life of the elderly. The policy should deal not only with the questions of the contemporary aged. Aging *per se* is not a reason for anything; an old person is simply the end result of an entire lifespan. The goal should be a meaningful lifespan for every individual.

5. One of the central issues is how to provide meaningful social roles for the elderly and how to help them in the maintenance of a positive self-image. Progress in these matters may require re-evaluation of basic philosophical attitudes about old age. Instead of labelling old people as old-fashioned and incompetent, they should be understood as a continuously developing social resource that is of value even to younger generations. Rather than reducing old people to medical and social problems, they should be redefined as multiple human beings who possess life experience and wisdom as a social inheritance to be passed on to the rest of society.

References

1. **Bourgeois-Pichat, J.** La science de la population au service de l'homme. *Conférence sur la science au service de la vie.* Vienna, Institut de la Vie, 1979.
2. *World population and its age-sex composition by country, 1950–2000. Demographic estimation and projection as assessed in 1978.* New York, United Nations, 1981.
3. **Amann, A.** *The status and prospects of the aging in Western Europe.* Vienna, European Centre for Social Welfare Training and Research, 1981 (Eurosocial Occasional Papers, No. 8).
4. **Carp, F.M.** Housing and living environment of older people. *In:* Binstock, R.H. & Shanas, E., ed. *Handbook of aging and the social sciences.* New York, Van Nostrand Reinhold, 1976, pp. 244–268.
5. *Die gesellschaftliche Reintegration älterer Menschen in Österreich.* Veröffentlichung des Bundesministeriums für Wissenschaft und Forschung. Vienna, Springer Verlag, 1976.
6. **Boalt, G. & Åhlund, O.** *Socialmedicinsk tidskrift,* **55**: 562–567 (1978).
7. **Dieck, M.** *Wohnen und Wohnumfeld älterer Menschen in der Bundesrepublik. Bedingungen des Wohnens älterer Menschen in der Bundesrepublik.* Schriftenreihe des Deutschen Zentrums für Altersfragen e.V. Alterns-Forschung für die Praxis. Band II. Heidelberg, 1979.
8. **Zarras, J.** Greece. *In:* Palmore, E., ed. *International handbook on aging.* Westport, CT, Greenwood, 1980, p. 172.
9. **Blaxter, M.** Social class and health inequalities. *In:* Carter, C.O. & Peel, J., ed. *Equalities and inequalities in health.* London, Academic Press, 1976, pp. 111–125.
10. **Chebotarev, D.F. et al.** Problems of health and position of the elderly in socialist countries of Eastern Europe. *Zeitschrift für Alternsforschung,* **36**: 437–472 (1981).
11. **Piotrowski, J.** Old people, bureaucracy, and the family in Poland. *In:* Shanas, E. & Sussman, M.B., ed. *Family, bureaucracy, and the elderly.* Durham, NC, Duke University Press, 1977, p. 165.
12. **Heikkinen, E. et al.** *Scandinavian journal of social medicine,* **4**: 71–74 (1976).
13. **Munnichs, J.M.A.** Linkages of old people with their families and bureaucracy in a welfare state, the Netherlands. *In:* Shanas, E. & Sussman, M.B., ed. *Family, bureaucracy, and the elderly.* Durham, NC, Duke University Press, 1977, pp. 92–116.
14. **Schmitz-Scherzer, R.** *Contributions to human development,* **3**: 127–136 (1976).
15. **Cutler, S.J.** *Journal of gerontology,* **32**: 470–479 (1977).
16. **Havighurst, R.J. et al.** *Adjustment to retirement. A cross-national study.* Assen, Van Gorcum, 1972.
17. **Graney, M.J.** *Journal of gerontology,* **30**:701–706 (1975).
18. **George, L.K.** *Journal of gerontology,* **33**: 840–847 (1978).
19. **Cutler, S.J.** *Journal of gerontology,* **31**: 462–470 (1976).
20. **Cunningham, D.A. et al.** *Journal of gerontology,* **23:** 551–556 (1968).

21. **Heikkinen, E.** Gerontological aspects of physical activity. *In*: Harris, R. & Frankel, L.J., ed. *Guide to fitness after 50.* New York, Plenum Press, 1977.
22. *Statistical yearbook of Finland, 1980.* Helsinki, Central Statistical Office of Finland, 1981.
23. **Myers, G.C.** *Gerontologist,* **18**: 441–448 (1978).
24. **Rosenwaike, I. et al.** *American journal of public health,* **70**: 1074–1080 (1980).
25. **Valkonen, T.** *Mortality trends and projections in four nordic countries.* Department of Sociology, University of Helsinki, 1982.
26. **Brückel, K.W.** Krankheit und Alter. *In: Grundzüge der Geriatrie.* Munich-Berlin-Vienna, Urban & Schwarzenberg, 1975.
27. **Kalimo, E. et al.** Health and health care of elderly population in Finland. *In: Geron XXII Yearbook 1978–79.* Helsinki, Societas Gerontologica Fennica, 1980, pp. 65–74.
28. **Ruikka, I. et al.** *Annals med. sci. Fenn.* Series A. V. Medica, 1966, p. 120.
29. **Bergener, M. et al.** *Die gesundheitliche und soziale Situation älterer Menschen in der Großstadt.* Schriftenreihe des Bundesministers für Jugend, Familie und Gesundheit. Band 74. Stuttgart, W. Kohlhammer, 1979.
30. **Svanborg, A. et al.** *Läkartidningen,* **77**: 3729–3786 (1980).
31. **Shanas, E. et al.** *Old people in three industrialized societies.* London, Routledge & Kegan Paul, 1978.
32. **Tornstam, L.** *Gerontologist,* **15**: 264–270 (1975).
33. **Amann, A.** On problems, trends, and measures. *In:* Amann, A., ed. *Open care for the elderly in seven European countries. A pilot study in the possibilities and limits of care.* Oxford, Pergamon Press, 1980.
34. **Chebotarev, D.F. & Sachuk, N.N.** *Journal of the American Geriatrics Society,* **27**: 49–57 (1979).
35. **Eitner, S.** *Zeitschrift für Alternsforschung,* **34**: 197–200 (1979).
36. **Coward, R.T.** *Gerontologist,* **19**: 275–282 (1979).
37. **Holmes, M.B. & Holmes, D.** *Handbook of human services for older persons.* New York, Community Research Applications, Inc., 1979.
38. *The ageing of populations and its economic and social implications.* New York, United Nations, 1956 (Population Studies, No. 26).
39. **Guilmot, P.** The demographic background. *In: Population decline in Europe. Implications of a declining or stationary population.* London, Edward Arnold, 1978.
40. **Rosenmayr, L. & Rosenmayr, H.** *Der alte Mensch in der Gesellschaft.* Hamburg, Reinbek, 1978.
41. *Report of the World Assembly on Aging.* New York, United Nations, 1982 (A/CONF. 113/31).

Part IV

Conclusions and recommendations

8

Conclusions and recommendations of the meeting held in Berne, 22–26 March 1982

The conclusions and recommendations of the participants at the meeting presented in this chapter have been ordered, as far as possible, according to the major age groups to which they pertain, in accordance with the programme and agenda. In a number of respects, however, this classification is artificial and some overlap is unavoidable. Thus, to the extent that health profiles at subsequent ages are determined by behavioural and environmental action at an earlier age, the state of health of an individual will be influenced by, or be dependent on, the preceding life history. Consequently, strategies aimed at improving health in a particular age group must transcend that group in so far as the precursors of illness occur at earlier ages. In addition, it was considered necessary to distinguish a section on recommendations of a more general, that is non-age-specific, nature.

General

Population policy

1. Demographically, most countries in the Region have reached a post-transitional stage, characterized by low mortality and low fertility. Many of these countries currently experience a below-replacement fertility level. The new demographic situation, characterized by the presence of a high proportion of the elderly in the population, and in some cases by declining population size, is causing increasing concern among a number of policy-makers. As far as the lengthening of life is concerned, this phenomenon should be welcomed as a remarkable achievement of applied science and the result of intensive efforts in social and health care policy. With regard to below-replacement fertility, however, a new equilibrium between fertility and mortality will eventually need to be established. As far as short-term targets in this respect are concerned, a consensus of opinion is probably premature. Here a variety of attitudes prevail, with some accepting and even welcoming a temporary decline, primarily for ecological and global reasons, while others are of the opinion that a replacement level should be restored as soon as possible. It is clear that the problem of population growth is rather

different, and consequently requires a completely different policy approach, in those countries of the Region where fertility is still comparatively high.

2. Whereas traditionally, quantitative population growth or growth control has been of primary concern to policy-makers in demographically post-transitional or even transitional societies, the orientation of policy ought to be directed more towards the qualitative aspects of human life, behaviour and living conditions.

Health and social policy

3. Governments should assume a greater responsibility for public health through appropriate health and social legislation and more active health promotion schemes. In some instances, difficulties have arisen in adapting health care and social services to the changing demographic structure. Too often, the health service and social infrastructures, staffing, and financial resources are rigidly maintained at levels that are inappropriate for, or not distributed according to, changing social and health care needs. Policy-makers should therefore seek to respond to changing demographic structures and population needs rather than to the demands and self-interests of health care and social establishments. Policy-makers should also take into account the long-term effects of demographic inertia; changing demographic behaviour has multigenerational effects that largely transcend the urgent, short-term societal problems.

Research

4. With regard to further research, several recommendations were made, most of which can be achieved with available human and financial resources, mindful, however, that a considerable reallocation, reorganization and reorientation of available means and manpower may be necessary.

5. Population scientists and health and social researchers should mutually broaden their scope and work in closer collaboration in order to improve policy-oriented research into the relationship between demographic behaviour, demographic structures, and health and social care. National population research institutes or comparable university or private research centres already exist in many European countries. It is recommended that the work of such population centres be made more interdisciplinary, thereby facilitating a more integrated biopsychosocial approach to the study of population and health.

6. Given the current shift in the causation of several demographic phenomena such as fertility, morbidity and mortality from biological and environmental factors towards sociocultural and behavioural determinants, it is recommended that social and behavioural research in the field of population and health be encouraged and strengthened.

7. In view of the observed or suspected role of socioeconomic status and other social and biological factors in morbidity and mortality, and the

absence of thorough knowledge about them in many countries, it is recommended that more attention be systematically paid to these problems in order to minimize differentials in ill health.

8. Further research is necessary on the health and social implications, especially for the family, of the dual roles that working women adopt.

9. Health and social services policies must take into account developments within the major age groups. Appropriate information to guide the formulation of such policies must be readily available. At the same time, there is a growing need for more information about the services required by specific age groups. This is particularly important for the elderly; there are marked differences in, for example, marital status and morbidity and mortality, between the elderly and the very elderly and between males and females.

10. In view of the increasing aging of populations, gerontological research should be strengthened and encouraged through the greater allocation of resources.

11. Since it cannot be expected that additional resources will be allocated for population and health statistics, available resources should be used more efficiently so as to better exploit the available data sources, to improve their quality (especially in the field of morbidity), to unify their codification — also with a view to interregional and international comparisons — and to facilitate the linkage of data from different sources.

The Young Population (0–19 Years)

12. The simultaneous decline in mortality and fertility have led to a relative decrease in the proportion of young people below 20 years of age, with the exception of countries in the far south of the Region. There is no evidence to suggest that this trend or situation will change dramatically in the near future. However, this is not to imply that the problems peculiar to the young will diminish in extent or significance. On the contrary, serious efforts must be made to improve the health and social welfare of young people. Despite the good physical health which, on average, most young people now experience, the psychosocial demands on the individual of a complex technological society are increasing and must be addressed with more concern than hitherto.

Morbidity and mortality

13. Children are perceived more and more as a valuable and precious resource in society. Some morbidity and mortality is unavoidable, however, and efforts should be made to minimize its individual and societal effects, the prevention of disability being a priority area for such action.

14. Infant and childhood impairment should be reduced or avoided through genetic counselling before conception occurs, through antenatal

screening and care during pregnancy, and through a reduction in birth injuries. Antenatal, obstetric and paediatric services must be improved and, where necessary, reorientated to meet these objectives.

15. Among infants as well as adolescents, every effort must be made to avoid accidents and violence both inside and outside the home and to minimize their consequences.

16. The structure of various institutions (hospitals, schools, housing) should be adapted to meet the specific needs of the young disabled. At the same time, specific occupations should be created for them. Also, their families should be assisted to cope with the specific difficulties that these children encounter in their daily lives.

17. A regular component of the training of health and welfare personnel should be devoted to the specific problems of youth (smoking, alcoholism, drug use, early pregnancy, social relations).

Fertility and fertility regulation

18. Unplanned fertility among adolescents — which applies to a large majority of pregnancies in this age group — should be avoided, not only for biomedical reasons but also for reasons of later economic opportunity and family building. What is more, taking into consideration the increasing level of adolescent sexual activity and the lowering of the age at first sexual experience, it is imperative that adolescents are duly prepared for personal, sexual and family relationships and that sexual behaviour is accompanied by adequate contraceptive protection.

Education

19. The increasing gap between biological maturation, which occurs earlier, and social maturity, which is reached at later ages, as well as the continuous fundamental and apparently irreversible sociocultural changes and the individualistic behaviour of the young, ought to be given due consideration by the authorities in developing educational, health and social policies.

20. Educational and social programmes should be formulated and implemented so as to facilitate the integration of young people into active life. To this end, instruction in social and cultural roles should better equip them to deal with conflicts and to be more responsible in the use of their rights and in the performance of their duties within society.

21. The education of children and adolescents in matters of health, sexuality and psychosocial growth should be considered as fundamental elements of health and social policy for this age group. This must be complemented by adequate and parallel programmes to inform and educate the parents. To this end, the mass media could be widely used.

22. Societal education of the young merits full attention to ensure their full and creative participation in society and thus avoid the social evils (violence, drugs, etc.) that afflict youth in particular.

23. The professional training of educators should include instruction in the understanding, acceptance and proper handling of the disabled and other vulnerable groups of young people.

Family life

24. Increasing female employment requires additional child care resources from society. In addition to the considerable increase in the number of care facilities required (crèches, kindergartens, child-minders, etc.) the standard of these services with regard to such factors as food quality, and compatibility between activities in the home and the child care situation, must be borne in mind.

25. Special attention should be paid to the specific problems of children from broken homes, the number of whom is increasing, as well as to children of other single-parent families. The absence of a family structure may be prejudicial to the health and psychosocial welfare of the child. Adequate financial support to meet the needs of such children should be forthcoming and a matter of priority.

26. The integration of migrant children into the host society can be accompanied by particular health and cultural problems. Special health and social services may be necessary and adequate and acceptable cultural and educational programmes should be made available.

The Adult Population (20–59 Years)

27. The expected size of the adult population in Europe in the year 2000 is already known with reasonable certainty from demographic projections. This population size is unlikely to be much different from that of today. However, the age structure of this group will undoubtedly alter, with a higher proportion of older adults by the year 2000.

28. The elderly population in the year 2000 will be composed of the survivors of the adult population of today, which in turn depends on past fertility rates. These rates have been declining throughout the Region, with the exception of the countries in the far south. Thus it must be expected that the adult population in the year 2000 will have to bear a greater economic burden in their support of the elderly than has hitherto been the case.

Family formation

29. The trend towards smaller family and household size, coupled with increasing divorce rates, will lead to an increase in the number of adults living alone and in the number of single-parent families. This group generally not only has poorer health than a two-adult family, but also poses a special problem for the provision of institutional and social services for its health care. It is expected that the size of this group will increase, and consequently greater provision will be necessary to meet its health requirements.

30. It is recognized that forms of cohabitation other than legal marriage are becoming increasingly common. This will necessitate a greater flexibility in the provision of health and social services and, in certain countries, legal measures to cope with this situation.

31. Bearing in mind the universally accepted principle that couples have the right to choose freely and responsibly the number and spacing of their children, information should be made available to parents to the effect that risk factors for mothers and offspring increase at higher parities and that family size should not exceed a safe level. The implications of trends in contraceptive practices and abortion must be recognized by the educational system and the health profession with an appropriate allocation of health resources.

32. Attention should be focused on the implications of increasing rates of divorce and the changing divorce pattern in European countries, in view of the possible psychological problems that may follow family breakdown.

33. Trends in family composition have important implications for the provision of housing. The future needs of the various household composition types and their likely geographical placement should be anticipated and planned for accordingly.

Women's participation in the workforce

34. Given the trend towards higher economic participation among women, there is a need for increased flexibility in working conditions to allow couples greater freedom in deciding their respective economic participation and the timing of such activity during the working life. This should permit a more equitable sharing of household and parental responsibilities. Community education about the implications of changing female roles should be encouraged, especially among young men, and social incentives such as flexible pension schemes should be introduced to facilitate and accommodate these changes in the family life cycle.

Health trends

35. While the overall level of mortality among adults in the European Region is comparatively low, the recent trend has varied considerably from one country to another. In particular, adult male mortality in some countries has been increasing in recent years. Furthermore, marked differentials in ill health exist among population subgroups, leading to specific sectors of the population who are especially vulnerable and consequently suffer increased health risks. The health needs of these groups must be recognized, and appropriate and effective health promotion measures should be developed to reduce their risk. This may necessitate a non-traditional approach to health education.

36. There is substantial evidence that current health risks among adults are increasingly attributable to detrimental lifestyles. Individuals should be

encouraged and educated to assume greater responsibility for their own health. Furthermore, societal measures should be developed to modify the impact of harmful environmental influences so that such individual efforts become more realistic in promoting good health.

37. Governments should be encouraged to formulate in their health strategies specific health and social targets aimed at reducing the level of mortality and morbidity among adults due to detrimental lifestyles and harmful environmental influences.

38. More research is necessary on the comparative effectiveness of various programmes designed to reduce the level of ill health in the community.

39. Although not directly linked to demographic factors, unemployment (and especially extended unemployment) is recognized as an important factor having prejudicial consequences for health. Efforts should be made to provide greater support for the unemployed. Among others, the value of alternative social inputs should be more widely recognized.

Migration

40. The nature of the migration process in the European Region is generally well understood, with new arrivals typically moving directly to the centre of urban areas. Often these city centres are in a state of decline. Moreover, the migrant stock is unlikely to decrease in the near future at least. The special health and social needs of these migrant communities must be recognized, and appropriate and acceptable health and social services must be provided for their care in accordance with cultural traditions.

41. The immigration process itself is likely to alter the social structure within the host country. The volume, nature and distribution of health and social services should be planned accordingly.

42. Countries in the European Region are at different stages of urbanization. The process of internal migration must be monitored continuously and health and social services, including health personnel, should be distributed and, if necessary, relocated accordingly.

The Elderly Population (60 Years and Over)

Longevity

43. European societies are facing the prospect of an increasing population of elderly people with a longer expectation of life than ever before. These developments are to be welcomed. It is also encouraging that, in general, the younger age groups among the elderly will enjoy better standards of health and education than formerly. The rapid increase in the number of the very old will, on the other hand, increase the need for services in all spheres of social life.

44. Although society will undoubtedly face new problems as a result of these developments, it is important to consider the aging process as a normal development which in itself need not be problematic. European societies must be prepared to face and cope with the challenges presented by the aging of their populations. It is essential to ensure that attitudes towards elderly people are such that the aging process comes to be increasingly regarded as an integrated part of the life cycle.

Retirement

45. A central issue is the provison of relevant social roles for the elderly. Too often, the attainment of retirement age implies exclusion from normal social life in which the working role is paramount. Clearly, this situation is problematic for many pensioners who wish to continue with their work and who are capable of doing so. However, other tendencies in favour of early retirement must also be borne in mind, the most prominent of which is the serious level of unemployment among younger people. It must be recognized, nonetheless, that the elderly constitute a potential resource which could be used for important tasks in society.

46. More flexible retirement policies should be developed. Among other aims, these should allow for part-time employment after normal retirement age. Occupational health measures and legislation should also be strengthened to reduce the differences in health status between occupational groups and to ensure a more equitable attainment of satisfactory retirement age. In combination with opportunities for retraining, such policies could conceivably help to reconcile some of the problems of the young and the older age groups.

Social isolation

47. Data from several countries show an increasing number of older people living alone, and this tendency is likely to continue. Contributory factors include smaller family size in the preceding generation and increased social mobility. Living alone does not necessarily imply social isolation, provided relatives and friends live close at hand and contact is maintained. Nevertheless, social isolation has adverse effects on the health of older people affected and renders the delivery of social and other services more difficult.

48. It would not be advisable, in most countries, to attempt to develop social policies aimed at reconstituting the extended family. More imaginative and appropriate social policies must be developed to reduce the social isolation of the elderly or, where possible, prevent its occurrence.

49. The search for relevant social roles in old age must begin before retirement. In some countries pre-retirement programmes have been introduced on an experimental basis to assist this process. These programmes should be encouraged and extended.

Policies for health and social services

50. Older people are heavy consumers of both health and social services. (One may note in passing that many older workers are obliged to retire early because of ill health and disability.) Appropriate health and social care must be available and readily accessible to the elderly, and means to ensure the delivery of such services should be developed where necessary.

51. Traditionally, great reliance has been placed on institutional care of the elderly. The cost of such hospital care is increasing and, moreover, many of the elderly who are institutionalized could equally well have received the necessary care in their homes.

52. In many countries agencies have been developed to meet the housing needs of the elderly; such agencies are adapted to their requirements for social care and support and for medical treatment. The work of these agencies needs to be effectively coordinated with a consequent strengthening of primary health care for the elderly.

53. Greater emphasis should be placed on improving the training of staff in all disciplines related to the needs of the elderly and on the coordination of services, so as to enable older people to retain their independence and remain in their own homes for as long as possible.

Education and training

54. The health and social situation of the elderly can also be improved by developing and strengthening education and training programmes. Considerable intercountry variation exists in the level of training of medical and social personnel in different fields of gerontology. This variation should be reduced so as to provide the professional groups concerned with adequate knowledge of, proper skills for, and correct attitudes towards treating the different problems of old age.

55. Educational programmes should also be developed for the elderly themselves to enable them to cope with activities in various spheres of life, and thereby to promote further opportunities for continuous self-development.

56. The public should be better informed about the aging process and the nature of old age. Information of this type could be provided by the mass media and should encourage a more positive attitude towards old people and their problems.

Annex 1

Participants

Ms E. Adams, Population Activities Unit, General Economic Analysis Division, Economic Commission for Europe, Geneva, Switzerland

Dr R. Beckers, Director-General, Ministry of Public Health and Family Affairs, Brussels, Belgium

Professor R.L. Cliquet, Centre for Population and Family Studies, Brussels, Belgium

Mr P. Gottely, Organization and Informatics Division, Ministry of National Solidarity, Paris, France

Dr S. Haberman, Head, Actuarial Science Division, The City University, London, United Kingdom

Professor E. Heikkinen, Department of Health Sciences, University of Jyväskylä, Finland

Mr L. Herberger, Director, Division of Population Statistics and Federal Institute of Population Research, Federal Statistical Office, Wiesbaden, Federal Republic of Germany

Dr L.B. Hunt, Senior Medical Officer, Department of Health and Social Security, London, United Kingdom

Dr A. Klinger, Chief, Demographic Statistics Department, Central Statistical Office, Budapest, Hungary

Mr G.J. Knaggs, Principal Administrator, Statistical Office, Commission of the European Communities, Luxembourg

Dr A. Leitao, Directorate-General of Health, Lisbon, Portugal

Mr C. Lindmark, Head, Planning and Statistical Department, National Board of Health and Welfare, Stockholm, Sweden

Mr C. Minder, Scientific Officer, Institute of Social and Preventive Medicine, Berne, Switzerland

Mr J.L. Murray, Administrative Officer, Secretary of the Steering Committee on Population, Council of Europe, Strasbourg, France

Mr J.E. Neury, Head, Division of Population Statistics, Federal Statistical Office, Berne, Switzerland

Professor S. Orzeszyna, Centre for Medical Postgraduate Education, Warsaw, Poland

Professor G. Papaevangelou, Athens School of Hygiene, Greece

Dr A. Rogers, Chairman, Human Settlements and Services Area, International Institute for Applied Systems Analysis, Laxenburg, Austria

Mr P. Schatzer, Information Officer, United Nations Fund for Population Activities, Geneva, Switzerland

Mr H. Seiler, Scientific Assistant, Federal Office of Public Health, Berne, Switzerland

Ms S. Teper, Department of Community Health, University Hospital and Medical School, University of Nottingham, United Kingdom

Professor T. Valkonen, Helsinki University Institute of Sociology, Helsinki, Finland

Mr K. van der Windt, Ministry of Health and Environmental Protection, Leidschendam, Netherlands

Mr M. Wyss, Scientific Officer, Federal Statistical Office, Berne, Switzerland